D1011445

THE RELIGION OF BEAUTY
IN WOMAN

THE RELIGION OF BEAUTY
IN WOMAN,

AND OTHER ESSAYS ON PLATONIC
LOVE IN POETRY AND SOCIETY,

BY

JEFFERSON BUTLER FLETCHER, *1865-1946*

Whatever fair is, is by nature good
— Spenser

HASKELL HOUSE
Publishers of Scholarly Books
NEW YORK
1966

PREFACE

THE following essays are chapters of a possible literary history of Woman. Written mostly by men, this *literary* history has treated, with curious alternation, its subject as idol or doll. Her influence has been held supermannish — daimonic or demonic — under the prevalence of ideals monastic, chivalric, or platonic; in the intervening moments of enlightenment, *Aufklarung*, common sense, she has — up to date — been dissected, and declared to be "stuffed with sawdust." With occasional and individual exceptions, she has apparently been contented to accept this masculine writing up — or down — of her spiritual significance. "The greater part of what women write about women," declared their champion, John Stuart Mill, "is mere sycophancy to men." Recently, perhaps, "we have changed all that;" possibly, no future Meredith will be justified in charging that

> Their sense is with their senses all mixed in,
> Destroyed by subtleties these women are!

"More brain" may, as he thinks, be coming to be their salvation — and ours; but the new concord of equality is still, as Byron says, subject to "the secret influence of the sex;" and while that lasts, Byron's further words ring warningly: —

> Alas! the love of women! it is known
>   To be a lovely and a fearful thing;
> For all of theirs upon that die is thrown,
>   And if 'tis lost, life hath no more to bring
> To them but mockeries of the past alone.

Mixed in tone and treatment as these essays are they do glance from various angles at one interesting event in the literary history of woman — the rise and fall of a peculiar worship, or maybe idolatry, of her physical and spiritual beauty as a means of grace. Of course, platonic love still lives in gentle hearts, however they be modern: while there is sex there is sentiment. But the ideal varies in color and fragrance with the social soil from which it springs. In these days, one is apt to designate as " platonic" a certain free-and-easy good-fellowship or ' chumminess' between men and women, veritably antipodal to the mystic aloofness of Dante's worship of Beatrice or even Michelangelo's austere veneration for Vittoria Colonna. Renaissance " platonic love" is indeed a complex thing, but it is simple at least in its spirit of aristocratic exclusiveness: for the 'gentle hearts' of gentle folk. As a "religion" it is 'high church,' ritualistic. It never can happen again — in precisely the same way.

Grateful acknowledgment is made to the *Atlantic Monthly*, *The Nation*, *The Dante Society*, and *Modern Philology* for their kind permissions to reprint certain of the essays in this volume.

TABLE OF CONTENTS

xi

THE RELIGION OF BEAUTY IN WOMAN

I suspect that my title may lead to a false impression. It seems to promise something of the ecstatic kind on which John Ruskin used to discourse. But really I mean the phrase, religion of beauty in woman, with prosaic literalness. I mean that in the Renaissance, in the later fifteenth century and after, there developed actually a kind of divine worship of beauty, and more especially of beautiful women. This "new religion" had its Peter, the rock on which it was founded, in Cardinal Pietro Bembo; its messiah, in Plato; its first and greatest commandment, in platonic love. The term "platonic love" has been spoiled for us. We smile at its mention. To our downright common sense, platonic love is wooden iron : it is either too nice to be platonic, or too platonic to be nice. Even in the Renaissance it too often meant something silly or worse. Bembo himself was no unspotted prophet; and some of the female "saints" of the "new religion" were as sepulchres but thinly whited. Yet a creed with such apostles as Castiglione, Michelangelo, Vittoria Colonna, Margaret of France, Philip Sidney, Edmund Spenser, John Donne, is not lightly to be scoffed away.

The creed took form in Italy.   Plato's idealism is behind it; but it is the passion for beauty of the Renaissance itself, and no mere metaphysical system, that gives fervor to the mood, is the soul within the doctrine.   The Italian of the Renaissance, however, was also an exceedingly concrete person; to parody Meredith, —

> *His* sense was with his senses all mixed in.

He meant by beauty, for all Plato, sensuous beauty, the beauty he could touch, see, hear, smell, taste.   From his passionate sensuousness derived his supremacy in the plastic arts, the pictorialism of his poetry, and its deficiency in imaginative suggestion.   Taking for granted that we are as much in love with the sensuously beautiful thing as he is, he spares us no detail of it.   In a pastoral allegory, the *Nymphal of Admetus*, Boccaccio describes seven charming nymphs, one after another.   They differ in type only as the superlatively beautiful differs from the supremely beautiful; yet we are treated to a complete list of specifications for each.   We feel at last like judges at a strange beauty-show.   But Boccaccio was justified of his own generation, and of some five generations more. Early in the fifteenth century, about 1430, Lorenzo Valla, who loved, like Mr. Bernard Shaw, to *épater le bourgeois*, wrote in Latin a dialogue *On Pleasure, or Concerning the True Good*. Pleasure, he says, is the true good; virtue for its own sake is an empty word. And the most pleasure-giving things are health and beauty, — especially beauty : for the more health we have, the less we know it; but the possession of beauty is a conscious joy forever. And of all beauty, best is the beauty of women. "What," he asks, "is sweeter, what more delectable, what more adorable, than a fair face?" And since beauty is not of the face merely, he would have beautiful women in summer go lightly clad, or clad not at all. It is an artist of the beautiful that speaks, not a voluptuary; only the man that hath no beauty in himself will misconceive him. "He that rejoices not in beauty, is blind either of soul or of body; and if he have eyes, they should be put out, for he knows not how to use them."

This absorbing passion for feminine beauty reveals itself everywhere. With Fra Lippo's wistful girl-faces it invades religious painting, before dominated by the hieratic, inaccessible, scarcely human type of Byzantine symbolists. And from Fra Lippo to Titian, Italian religious art is mostly a vision of fair women, labeled saints, madonnas, what you will, but conceived and valued as fair women. On April 15, 1485, as Burckhardt relates, an interesting thing happened. There was found in a marble sarcophagus on the Appian Way the body of a young Roman girl, so marvelously embalmed that she seemed alive. Her eyes were half open; her lips parted as if smiling; her cheeks rosy. The body was laid in state in a palace on the Capitol. All flocked to look, painters among the rest; "for," says the chronicler, "she was more beautiful than can be said or written, and, were it said or written, it would not be believed by those who had not seen her." Very likely all this did not happen quite as it is reported for us; but that does not matter. The interesting thing is, that whereas their grand-fathers would have worshiped this seeming resur-rection as miracle, or anathematized it as witch-craft, these artists of the Renaissance prostrated themselves before a miracle indeed — the miracle of a pretty woman!

While Italian hearts were warming to this particular kind of miracle, two things came to pass which focused their diffused sentiment to a prac-tical end, and justified this practical end to the intelligence. I mean the rehabilitation of Plato, and the social emancipation of women.

Plato had not been without influence, indeed, during the earlier Christian period or the Middle Ages. From Augustine to Gerson, on the contrary, his thought had impregnated Christian doctrine. But from the ninth century to the fifteenth, the authority of his rival, Aristotle, was absolute, dwarfing every other human authority whatsoever. Aristotle was not only, as Dante hailed him, "master of them that know," he was also preceptor of them that would be saved. To reconcile faith and reason, Thomas Aquinas found it sufficient to reconcile faith and Aristotle. Aristotle was the adopted *doctor evangelicus* of the Christian Church; Plato remained a mere pagan philosopher.

First to protest against this medieval order of precedence is Francis Petrarch. In his *Triumph of Fame*, Plato walks before Aristotle : —

I turned me to the left, and Plato saw,
Who in that troop came nearest to the goal
Towards which they strive who gifted are of God.
Next Aristotle full of genius high . . .

And elsewhere Petrarch notes that Plato appeals to princes and potentates, Aristotle to the vulgar herd : *Ego arbitror quod inter duos, quorum alterum principes proceresque, alterum universa plebs laudat.*

In the fifteenth century the issue thus raised

became an all-absorbing interest. The center of dispute was Florence; and Plato's partisans were, in the first instance, prominent Greeks drawn there by the patronage of Cosmo de' Medici, or attendant upon their Emperor John Palæologos, when he came to discuss with the Roman Pope a possible harmonization of East and West in faith. Out of the interest in Plato, revived by these Greeks, grew the so-called Platonic Academy of Florence, of which the leading spirits were Marsilio Ficino and young Giovanni Pico della Mirandola. These two men devoted their learning and talents to the reconciliation of faith and reason; but for them no longer Aristotle, but Plato, sums all that reason can. Plato's triumph is complete; he is now the *doctor evangelicus* whom Ficino preaches in the Church of the Angels in Florence. "Within this church we would expound the religious philosophy of our Plato. We would contemplate divine truth in this seat of Angels. Enter in, dear brethren, in the spirit of holiness." And Ficino's later patron, Lorenzo de' Medici, adds the practical sanction, "Without the Platonic, discipline, no one can be either a good citizen, or a good Christian."

But Plato's doctrines were given a markedly mystic significance by these Florentines, fresh from the Church Fathers, vitally interested in the metaphysics of love of Dante and his circle, drawn, above all, to the dreamy speculations of the half-oriental Plotinus. These side influences tended to make paramount in their new religion that element of platonism which finds chief utterance in the *Symposium:* that love is the supreme force, cosmic, moral, religious; that there are two loves, heavenly and earthly, the one a desire of the beauty of sense, the other a desire of the beauty above sense; and that, as sensuous beauty is the shadow of supersensuous or spiritual beauty, therefore by following the shadow we may ultimately attain to the reality behind the shadow, and in an ecstasy possess divine beauty itself.

Thus fatally, as if by preëstablished harmony, this whole body of exotic doctrine came to sanction and codify the mastering instinct of these beauty-loving Florentines, avatars in so many traits of Plato's own people. But like the Greeks themselves, the Florentines, much as they might speculate upon the supremacy of abstract beauty, the beauty visible only to the mind's eye, actually responded how much more sincerely, passionately, to concrete beauty, beauty visible to the eye of sense. To a few, in moments of speculative exaltation, this earthly beauty might dissolve away to the shadow their creed declared it to be; but to most of them, in effect, the visible, tangible, audible shadow was the reality they loved, whether purely or impurely. Yet contemplation of beauty, living with beauty, as a moral tonic, a discipline of excellence, might indeed be sincerely realized and fervently advocated, even by men-of-the-world for whom mystic passion for a supersensuous ideal was, though not necessarily mere shamming, yet an emotional state of which they were by temperament incapable altogether, or capable only in rare passing moods.

Any one conversant with the character of Lorenzo the Magnificent, for instance, would hardly credit him with more than a verbal comprehension of any mystic passion.   I do not mean because he was a man of loose morals : a man may feel, as well as see, the better, and yet follow the worse.   I mean that Lorenzo's temperament was too exclusively Latin, too clear-sighted, logical, positive.   Yet we have no reason to doubt his sincerity when he urged the moral efficacy of love against any who might censure his love-poetry as vain and amatorious writing.   He argues with the calm leisureliness of a despot ; we need but note his conclusion, that excellent next to the love of God is that "rare kind of love" which is of one person and for always.   And such love cannot be unless the beloved "possess, humanly speaking, highest perfection ; and unless there be met to-

gether in her, besides physical beauty, a lofty intelligence, modest and refined habits and ways,
elegant mien and manners, suavity in address
and winning speech, love, constancy, and faith."

Lorenzo but seems to say long what Goethe
said short in

> Das Ewigweibliche
> Zieht uns hinan.

There is, however, an important difference.   For
Goethe the potency of the *Ewigweibliche* is all in
"love, constancy, and faith;" for the rest, his
Gretchen is a simple, unlettered village girl.
Such a priestess of love did not exist for the despot
of Florence and his fellow-platonists.   As little
would ancient Romans have thought of choosing
a vestal from the kitchen.   For the Renaissance,
das Ewigweibliche came at times perilously near
being translatable into the Everladylike.   "Love,
constancy, and faith" are part of her theoretical
equipment; but in Lorenzo's list, they tail off his
specifications rather weakly after his emphasized
particularity anent the social graces, the perfec-
tions of the inner circle, the salon.   Petrarch was
prophetic when he said that Plato was the philosopher for "princes and potentates;" in the
Renaissance the priestess of platonic love was the
fine lady.   She was the Everwomanly; the rest

were practicable females. The young platonist, Edmund Spenser, under the exigencies of the pastoral manner, called his "Rosalind" a shepherdess and a "widow's daughter of the glen;" but, lest we forget even for a moment, his confidential editor makes haste to reassure us that the convenances have not really been violated. "He calleth Rosalind the Widowes daughter of the glenne, that is of a country Hamlet or borough, which I thinke is rather sayde to coloure and concele the person, then simply spoken. For it is well knowen, even in spighte of Colin and Hobbinoll, that shee is a Gentlewoman of no meane house, nor endewed with anye vulgare and common gifts, both of nature and manners: but such indeede, as neede nether Colin be ashamed to have her made knowen by his verse, nor Hobbinol be greved that so she should be commended to immortalitie for her rare and singular vertues."

If we are curious to know just what the Renaissance thought of when it described a lady as not "endewed with anye vulgare and common gifts, both of nature and manners," there are at hand dozens of contemporary books to enlighten us. The sixteenth century was indefatigable in its eagerness to define, to form, and to inform its lady worthy to be loved. It measured her from top to toe; it put the right words into her mouth;

it scaled to a hair-line the boundary between coquetry and *cocotterie*. Among others, Messer Angelo Firenzuola sets her physical type with accuracy. (I condense for convenience from Burckhardt's summary.) "Her hair should be a soft yellow, inclining to brown; the forehead just twice as broad as high; skin transparent, not dead white; eyebrows dark, silky, most strongly marked in the middle, and shading off toward the ears and nose; the white of the eye faintly touched with blue, the iris not actually black, but soft deep brown; the lids white, and marked with almost invisible tiny red veins; the hollow round the eye of the same color as the cheek; the ear, of a medium size, with a stronger color in the winding than in the even parts, with an edge of the transparent ruddiness of the pomegranate; the nose to recede gently and uniformly in the direction of the eyes; where the cartilage ceases, there may be a slight elevation, but not so marked as to make the nose aquiline; the lower part to be less strongly colored than the ears, but not of a chilly whiteness, and the middle partition above the lips to be lightly tinted with red; the mouth smallish, neither projecting to a point, nor quite flat, with lips not too thin, and fitting neatly together; except in speaking or laughing never more than six upper teeth should be displayed.

As points of finesse may pass a dimple in the upper lip, a certain fullness of the lower lip, a tempting smile in the left corner of the mouth." And so on; for our connoisseur continues his minuscular analysis incorrigibly to the bitter end, — and with gravity, for to him there are sermons in looks.

Others delineate with similar particularity the spiritual woman. Count Baldassare Castiglione is the most worth listening to; for it is his gentleman and his lady, as characterized in the *Libro del Cortegiano*, that European high life in the sixteenth century labored to reproduce and in some measure did reproduce. According to Castiglione, the soul of gentility in man or woman is *grazia*, grace. At bottom, grace is the trained instinct which can do or say difficult things with apparent ease. In the lady, grace involves moreover *una certa mediocrità difficile*, "a certain golden mean of unapproachableness." Her demeanor should spell the maxim —

> Be bolde, be bolde, and everywhere be bolde
> *   *   *   *   *   *   *
> Be not too bolde!

No timid shrinking Gretchen she, but skilled in "a certain pleasing affability," and adept in *ragionamenti d'amore*, "conversings of love," which "every gentle sir uses as means to acquire grace with ladies . . . not only when impelled by passion, but often as well to do honor to the lady with whom he speaks, it seeming to him that the pretence of loving her is a testimony of her worthiness to be loved." So gently courted, she will, while she can, "seem not to understand;" or, that ruse failing, will "take all as a merry jest." Singing, playing, dancing, — all social accomplishments must be in her repertory of fascination; but she must not be forthputting in them, rather, after a not excessive pressing, should yield "with a certain coyness" (*con una certa timidità*).

Enough: we begin to recognize her, this fine lady of the Italian Renaissance. She is a work of art, of a subtle artistry

That nature's work by art can imitate.

The natural woman is to her as the rough-hewn block to the finished statue. She could apprehend with enthusiasm Keats's apothegm, "Beauty is truth;" but she would have shrugged her powdered shoulders at the complementing, "Truth beauty." In her pragmatic way she identified truth with tact. No doubt the ladies of Castiglione's generation had quite too robust nerves to be altogether precious dolls. We hear how Isabella of Este used to put on the gloves with her pretty cousin, Beatrice, and once with a clever counter floored her. Despite Castiglione's protest against such "strenuous and rough mannish sports," the term "virago" was not yet one of contumely : Britomart the bold had her votaries as well as Amoret the amiable ; but none the less, eighteenth-century Belinda is already in sight, — Belinda, whose "little heart" but turns to thoughts of beaux, and whose

Awful Beauty puts on all its arms

to conquer — Sir Fopling Flutter !

It was a recognition, just if partial, of this manifest tendency in the Renaissance "religion of beauty," artificial beauty, that drew from moral John Ruskin many a tirade. "All the Renaissance principles of art tended," he exclaims, "as I have before often explained, to the setting Beauty above Truth, and seeking for it always at the expense of truth. And the proper punishment of such pursuit — the punishment which all the laws of the universe rendered inevitable — was, that those who thus pursued beauty should wholly lose sight of beauty. . . . The age banished beauty, so far as human effort could succeed in doing so, from the face of the earth, and the form of man. To powder the hair, to patch the cheek, to hoop

the body, to buckle the foot, were all part and
parcel of the same system which reduced streets
to brick walls, and pictures to brown stains. One
desert of ugliness was extended before the eyes of
mankind; and their pursuit of the beautiful, so
recklessly continued, received unexpected con-
summation in high-heeled shoes and periwigs, —
Gower Street and Gaspar Poussin." This is
perhaps like judging apples ripe by apples rotten;
yet it does nevertheless put finger on a rotten
spot in the Renaissance passion for beauty.

But I digress too far. In my effort to picture
the ideal "beauty" of the period as she was, and
as she threatened to become, I have forgotten
our present concern with her, namely, how her
emergence acted upon the platonic cult, and how
she in turn was reacted upon by that cult.

The story of her emergence itself can here only
be hinted at. The woman of the earlier fifteenth
century, even in Italy, was, so far as social activity went, still in the kindergarten stage. Luther,
who in this respect remained obstinately old-
fashioned, expressed the earlier Italian view of her
whole duty, when he said in his *Table Talk*,
"Take women out of the household, and they are
good for nothing. . . . Woman is born to keep
house, it is her lot, her law of nature." Unhappily for such masculine ruling, however, woman

has shown at several periods of her history a disposition — and a faculty — for overruling this particular law of her nature. She has uniformly appealed to another law, equally of her nature, which went into operation with Adam. *"The woman tempted me;"* and so Adam yielded to the woman — against his better judgment. So long as Luther can keep his woman in the household, that "law of nature" of hers is safe. Luther also is safe, — as a bird is safe from a serpent inexperienced in fascination. But the instinct and the power are there, and on provocation may grow dangerous.

In this fifteenth-century Italy, woman's provocation came in the form of the higher education, the awakening and training of that *"ingegno grande,"* that "lofty intelligence," which Lorenzo de' Medici found so essential to the ideal loved one. The wisdom of the serpent was once more to subjugate man. The new learning, based as it was upon *belles lettres*, appealed to girlish minds. The old scholastic régime of logic and dialectic, if it reached them at all, hardened and unsexed them; but the new literature warmed their imaginations, touched their sympathies, lubricated their tongues. Tales of precocious maids becoming, while still in their teens, accomplished orators, poets, scholars in Latin, even in Greek,

go the rounds of Italy. Teachers, pleased and
flattered, egg on their pupils to emulation. The
femme savante appears. If she is high-born and
rich and ambitious, she sets up her salon. There
she can meet men on equal terms, for wit and
learning; and, if she happens to be a pretty woman also — well, Luther and all his "laws of
nature" cannot put her back into the household
to stay. The odd thing is that these very human-
ists, who were so largely responsible for letting
woman out of the household, were all the while
theoretically urging the necessity of keeping her
in there. One of the foremost of them, Leo
Battista Alberti of Florence, in his famous *Treatise
on the Family*, draws his ideal girl-bride meekly
making obeisance to her husband. "She told
me," this lordly personage remarks, "that she had
learned to obey her father and mother; and had
received their injunction always to obey me; and
accordingly was prepared to do whatever I might
command." Yet it was good Leo Battista and his
kind who were responsible for Beatrice, the girl-
let-out-of-the-household, answering Benedick's
pathetic "Do you not love me?" with her "Why,
no; no more than reason. . . . I would not deny
you; but, by this good day, I yield upon great
persuasion; and partly to save your life, for I
was told you were in a consumption."

c

Now, by the end of the fifteenth century, Beatrice was become for Italy a fact, the paramount fact, socially speaking. In the person of Castiglione's Emilia Pia — first cousin moral of Beatrice — mad and merry wit rules it over the brilliant group in the salon at Urbino; she and Signor Gasparo "never meet but there's a skirmish of wit between them." To such clever women, sure of themselves and so daring much, the new Renaissance literature is being dedicated and devoted. Their influence is in all and over all, making for social rightness and mostly — it is fair to say — for righteousness. There is no longer question of their right to influence men, but only what to do with that influence, how to direct it, and to what end. And Pietro Bembo, *élégant* and poet, theologian and wit, is ready with an answer, blending metaphysics with gallantry, with a spice of anti-matrimonial cynicism. This last, this odium attaching to marriage, came to the Renaissance from several quarters of influence: from the practical and theological arguments of the Fathers, especially Ambrose and Augustine, against marriage; from the fanatic asceticisms of morbid Eastern anchorites, and their monkish disciples in the West; from the fantastic code of thirteenth-century chivalric love, with its statute as redacted by Chaplain Andrew, — *Dicimus enim et stabilito tenore firmamus amorem non posse inter duos jugales suas extendere vires:* "we say and legally resolve that love cannot extend its dominion over two joined in matrimony;" from the interminable line of travesties on marriage from Jean de Meung on; from the idealism of Guinicelli and Cavalcanti and Dante, and the sentimentalism of Petrarch; from, finally, Plotinus of Alexandria, next revered after Plato, who, without exactly condemning marriage, yet commends as the higher love that which rests in passionless contemplation of womanly beauty.

But although Plotinus emphasizes the virtue of such contemplative love, he is far from making feminine beauty its principal object. His conception of beauty, on the contrary, is more abstract even than Plato's. Nor were the earlier Florentine platonists, Ficino, Pico, Benivieni, and the rest, thinking of feminine beauty as the supreme beauty this side heaven. Lorenzo carefully distinguished between Plato's divine love, which is the highest good, and love for a human creature, which is a good only after a finite manner of speaking. But Cardinal Bembo, in *Gli Asolani*, definitively identifies platonic love with love of ladies, finds man's *summum bonum*, as Browning put it playfully, "in the kiss of one girl." In Bembo's philosophy there was indeed much virtue in a kiss.

In a fair garden of the Queen of Cyprus at
Asolo, three highborn maidens and as many
youths while away the hour of siesta with talk of
love. As the custom was, they elect one of the
maidens to preside over their debate. One of
the youths, Perottino, as "devil's advocate,"
attacks love, adducing many plausible reasons
why love should be held dangerous and hurtful,
occasion of many ills. Whereupon another youth,
Gismondo, defends love, matching each and every
allegation of ill by a joy won through loving; so
that, whereas Perottino concluded love to be
wholly bad, Gismondo proves love to be wholly
good. Both cannot be right; so the queen calls
upon Lavinello, the third youth, to break, if
possible, the deadlock. Love, he replies, is good
or bad according to its object; the object of the
love which is good is beauty alone. True beauty
man perceives through eye and ear and mind;
through these come those immortal harmonies
which delight and do not pall. Desire which is
not of such beauty is but

Expense of spirit in a waste of shame.

Such is the practical gist of Bembo's elegant
sermon, — stripped of the graces of style, the
poetry, the eloquence, lavished by the courtly
churchman. It was this gist that these culti-

vated, enthusiastic, ambitious ladies of the Renaissance took to heart, and made practical trial of. Bembo's book was to them what *La Nouvelle Héloïse* was to the ladies of French salons three centuries later, — a more intimate bible. And presently they were to hear the "Matthew Arnold" of that day actually substituting this new gospel according to Peter of Venice for the old gospel of Peter of Galilee.

Bembo's *Asolani* was published in 1505. During the winter of that year the conversation was supposed to take place which Castiglione records in his *Libro del Cortegiano*. The book is an epitome of the cultivated life, touching and illustrating every function of that life from boudoir and drawing-room to cabinet and throne. Last of all, and highest function of all, is naturally religion. And here, at the close of the book, where we might expect an exhortation to Christian love, we find instead an apostrophe to platonic love. Bembo himself is the officiating priest; and when at the last he comes down from the ecstatic vision he has himself evoked, he is like Moses returned from Sinai: "He seemed as if transported and spellbound, and stood mute and immobile, his eyes turned heavenward, as if he were distraught; until the Lady Emilia . . . took him by the hem of his garment, and plucking it gently, said,

'Have a care, Messer Pietro, lest with these thoughts your own spirit be reft away from the body.' — 'Madam,' replied Messer Pietro, 'nor would that be the first miracle which love hath worked in me.'"

Here in a single situation is the keynote of nearly all, — in truth a discordant note, sounding, or pretending to sound, high piety and light gallantry at once and in one. Ruskin is in so far right: the Renaissance religion of beauty started wrong. Whatever truth may lie in the notion of the platonic "ladder of love," the way towards the supra-mundane is unlikely to pass through the salon of *la grande mondaine*.

Still, however crossed at birth by a malignant spirit of levity, there is truth and beauty in Castiglione's ideal itself. "Who does not know," he asks, "that women cleanse our hearts of all evil and low thoughts, of cares, of troubles, and of those heavy dejections that follow in the train of these? And if we consider well, we shall recognize also, that in respect to the knowledge of high things, so far from turning away men's minds, women rather awaken them." Upon this faith as a cornerstone Castiglione builds his theory of the state. God has deputed the government of peoples to princes; princes should lean upon wise counsellors, mature enough in years to have out-

lived their own misguided passions, but fresh in
spirit to feel and follow the perfecting influence of
beauty.   The function of women in society, therefore, is by their beauty, of body and mind con-
joined, to lead upward and onward such men.
The Middle Ages, the age of Aristotle, had called
woman *confusio hominis*, the "confusion of man;"
the Renaissance, the age of Plato, now hailed her
in effect as *illuminatio Dei*, "the illumination of
God."   So Michelangelo : —

> From highest stars above
>   Downward a radiance flows,
>   Drawing desire to those;
> And here men call it love.

It was as if the mood of such men, like a prism,
refracted the figure of Mary, dearer divinity of
medieval Christendom, into many gracious and
beneficent living images, before each one of which
men might kneel and say, as Michelangelo himself to Vittoria Colonna, —

Rough-cast, first was I born . . .
From that rough cast of me, this better Me
From thee had second birth, thou high pure one.

She sustains him : —

Blest spirit, who with ardent earnestness,
My heart, aging towards death, keepest in life.

To her he prays: —

Lord of me, at the last hour
Reach out unto me thy two pitiful arms;
Take me from myself, and make me one to please thee.

Through her is salvation: —

Blessed the soul where runs no longer time
Through the permitted to contemplate God.

But on few descended the "radiance of the
stars" as on this magnificent old man, so voicing
his spiritual love at past sixty-three.   Castiglione
had indeed said "that old men can love blamelessly
and more happily than young; by this word 'old'
meaning indeed not decrepit, nor when the bodily
organs are so weak that the soul cannot longer
exercise its functions through them, but when
wisdom in us is in its fullness."   Michelangelo
justifies the opinion; and so, from the other side,
does Sir Philip Sidney, whose illumination from his
Star, Stella, is shot through with the smoky passions of undisciplined youth.   For long he cannot
find peace in the platonic — or shall we say
sisterly — love Stella offers him: —

Service and Honour, Wonder with Delight,
    Fear to offend, will worthy to appear,
Care shining in mine eyes, Faith in my sprite:
    These things are left me by my only Dear.
But thou, Desire! because thou wouldst have all,
Now banisht art: but yet, alas, how shall?

Yet he too at the last professes conversion in his sonnet, —

Leave me, O love, which reachest but to dust!

Beyond question, few converts to the Renaissance religion of beauty stood on the heights with Michelangelo and Sidney. Most of these — most who were professional poets, at any rate — remained in the comfortable valleys of patronage. For instance, Dr. John Donne writes to Lucy Harrington, Countess of Bedford: —

You have refined me, and to worthiest things. . . .

Yet to that deity which dwells in you,
Your virtuous soul, I now not sacrifice;
These are petitions, and not hymns. . . .

"Petitions, and not hymns" most of such tributes were. And Dr. Donne's list of "worthiest things" to which he has been "refined" — "virtue, art, beauty, fortune" — leads by its order of climax to the disquieting doubt that "Madam" has been dear to him less as Saint Beauty than as Saint Bounty. Indeed, too many a poet of the sixteenth century was a pilgrim to the latter's shrine; his platonic patron saint achieved sainthood only in the degree of her good works — *toward him*. Poets had to live; paying public there was none; so they borrowed from patrons and repaid with thanks keyed to the high pitch of spiritual love. Especially adapted for such amorous notes-of-hand was the sonnet as Petrarch wrote it, — a form brief, ingenious, pointed, pithy, a style all tender, obsequious, yet within bounds, delicate, a passion which flattered without compromising, in fine, a strictly legal currency for all compliment, or, in the platonic manner of speaking, a hymnal for the "new religion in love." Strange to say, the aptest description of Petrarch's love-poetry as conceived by the salon is by uncouthly pedantic Gabriel Harvey, Spenser's friend: "Petrarch was a delicate man, and with an elegant judgment graciously confined Love within the terms of Civility." His poetry is "the grace of Art, a precious tablet of rare conceits, and a curious frame of exquisite workmanship; nothing but neat Wit, and refined Elegance." Do we not hear, and see, the *petit maître* of the salon! Petrarch wrote of himself, —

> And I am one who find a joy in tears.

His mendicant followers reduced his stock of sentiment to sweet water, cooking this into sonnets of sugar-candy; and too many a "Sacharissa" was by nature, as well as by name, as Dr. Johnson said, "derived from sugar." Until John Cleveland might well cry out, —

> For shame, thou everlasting wooer . . .
> For shame, you pretty female elves,
> Cease thus to candy up yourselves!

The platonic religion of beauty far from died out with the Renaissance. It was given finical propagation during the early seventeenth century throughout Europe. Preciously modish in the *Hôtel de Rambouillet*, it was thence grafted afresh upon English high society by Henrietta Maria, full alumna of the French school. In Italy, meanwhile, it had degenerated into the silly institution of the *cicisbeo*, or platonic "servant," who was attached to every fashionable matron. Byron has drawn his portrait in *Beppo:*

> . . . "Cavalier Servente" is the phrase
> Used in politest circles to express
>   This supernumerary slave who stays
> Close to the lady as a part of dress,
>   Her word the only law which he obeys.
> His is no sinecure, as you may guess;
>   Coach, servants, gondola, he goes to call,
> And carries fan and tippet, gloves and shawl

The *cicisbeo* was regularly picked out, along with the husband, by the lady's family; and was supposed to exercise a kind of spiritual influence over her, untainted by the material bondage of matrimony.

As was natural, the platonic fashion spread

downward from the court.   Molière's *précieuses ridicules* and *femmes savantes* are of the *bourgeoisie.* We catch echoes of the *cicisbeo* even in England, and as late as Sheridan.   "You know," protests innocent young Lady Teazle to insinuating Joseph Surface, "I admit you as a lover no farther than fashion requires." — "True," replies Joseph, — "a mere Platonic cicisbeo, what every wife is entitled to." — "Certainly," assents the ingenuous lady, "one must not be out of the fashion."

The breaking down of such fashions was undoubtedly one of the many reactions against the artificial and unnatural, which, taken together, we call the Romantic Movement.   Castiglione's *Cortegiano* was the gospel of the Renaissance religion of beauty; the gospel of the Romantic religion of passion was Rousseau's *La Nouvelle Héloïse.* Rousseau swept away the whole code of gallant fencing, of suprasensuous ecstasies, of artificial courtesies; he took his lovers out of doors, out of overheated salons, not into smug gardens of trimmed box and simpering marbles, but into the presence of real nature, and real human nature, even if a little overwrought; and the fine fantastical French ladies and their beribboned gallants sighed over his pages and, even while remaining fine fantastical ladies and beribboned gallants, at least played at being ingenuous children of nature.

It would be interesting to trace the development from these play children of nature, these masqueraders in *fêtes galantes*, of the real child of nature, the ideal woman-type of the Romanticists. It would be interesting again to set beside the Renaissance belle, mistress of herself and men, shaving her forehead to appear intellectual, and graduating Connoisseur in Hearts, — to set beside her the Romantic heroine, Virginie, Dorothea, Gretchen, Cythna, Haidee, and all their sisters of drama and fiction, — innocent children, artless and helpless, who can only love, and, when their love is hurt, can only pine away with it, like Shelley's *Sensitive Plant*. One might also show reaction on reaction, and illustrate the child-woman of Goethe growing into the "interesting matron," *la femme de trente ans*, of Balzac and George Sand; or illustrate occasional reversion in our own time to the platonic ideal itself, as in the apostrophe of Jane in *L'ami des Femmes* of Dumas *fils*. "Let us forget earth," she sighs, "let us realize heaven; let us share our thoughts, our joys, our griefs, our aspirations, our tears, so that in this unfleshly communion of minds and souls there may be in our eyes pride, in our heart-throbs purity, in our speech chastity, in our consciences calm." So history — and women — repeat themselves. But all this would be another story.

DANTE AND BEATRICE

A Variety of Religious Experience

The definition of poetry as a "criticism of life" may be unhappily phrased, but its intention is sound. I doubt the dictum of Keats: a thing merely of beauty is not a sufficing joy forever. We have other than æsthetic emotions, other than emotional interests; and unless these also find their satisfaction in a poem, we are not, I think, wholly content with it. A supreme poem would respond to our whole nature; and in responding, reveal the poet's experience and judgment of life.

Dante's poetry is certainly, by this test, supreme. But while we cannot deny his many-sided responsiveness, we may perhaps question the significance of his responses for us. He looked at the world through glasses that no longer fit our eyes. Seen through them, life loses its accustomed perspective, and ordinary experience takes on prismatic colors which make it beautiful, but strange; so that out of his book of life we accept the poetry; the reality we question, or explain

30

away.   Most of all, we question, or explain away,
the reality of his experience of love ; that too must
be reckoned as "poetry," which, if not merest
allegory, seems at most an idealization as slightly
in touch with reality as a toy-balloon tied to the
ground by a thread.

Are we then, after all, reduced to the option of
reading Dante as the, for us, idle dreamer of a
day, not empty indeed, but past and gone, or as
the diarist of men and things once, but no longer,
living?   Does he appeal only to our antiquarian
and æsthetic sides?   Did he speak more literally
than he knew when he gave thanks solely for

> The good style, that has brought me honor ?

We live in an empirical age ; and the Prag-
matist appears to be its prophet.   Our test of
reality, of truth, is human experience ; and the
highest truth for us is that which, verified by
human experience, is of deepest import to humanity.   We are, as Newman said, not to be converted
by syllogisms : not that we need distrust reason,
but that we know every nexus of deduction to
depend ultimately upon a major premise unde-
duced and undeducible — save from experience.
Supernatural revelation, even were we personally
its recipients, would be discounted by us, because
we know too well the possibilities of self-illusion,

self-suggestion. But if a revelation were given to us, not supernatural, not alien to common experience, but verifiable therein, and of deepest import to humanity, assuredly we should be concerned to listen. And it is precisely such a revelation, I think, that Dante gives.

The one poem, of which the *New Life* and the *Divine Comedy* are parts, is the record of a religious experience. Its first crisis came in Dante's ninth year of age, when he first saw Beatrice, and heard in his heart the words, *Ecce deus fortior me.* The spiritual outcome of the experience is told in the last words of the *Divine Comedy:* —

> To the high fantasy here power failed ;
>   But already my desire and will were turned —
>   Even as a wheel revolving evenly —
> By the Love that moves the sun and other stars.

Such is the redeemed soul ; and of such is the kingdom of heaven. There the individual desire and will are not annihilated, not denied, but rather fulfilled ; for if one really desires and wills only what omnipotence wills, there can be no disappointment. Such an one is able to say in sincerity with the blessed,

> In His will is our peace.

Spontaneous self-surrender to the will of God is the goal of Dante's spiritual journey. Look-

ing backward along the way, he was able to see
the impulse to such surrender in his childish love;
and writing the story long after the event, he could
read into the mood of the child an intelligence
beyond the capacity of any child. *Ecce deus
fortior me:* it is "*lo spirito della vita*," the spirit
of life, the vital instinct of self, that is made to
speak; therefore it is no violence to translate
modernly, — Behold a god, Love, stronger than I,
who am the instinct of self.   And the occasion of
this self-overcoming impulse, Beatrice, is forthwith recognized as his "*beatitudo*," or blessedness,
not for the delight she may give, but for the spirit
of self-renunciation she calls forth.   Thus the
two extremes of his experience meet in one religious
mood; the child is no otherwise moved by the
little maiden than the man

By the love that moves the sun and other stars.

She is for him from the beginning the mouthpiece
of God, and the means of salvation.

There is nothing abnormal, nothing mystical,
in the situation.   The instinctive altruism of love
is no theory, but a fact of experience.   Any small
boy who, unintimidated, resigns the core of his
apple to another small boy feels it after his fashion.
Nancy Sykes dumbly devoted to her abominable
Bill; the rake of de Musset's poem suddenly piti-

D

ful of his poor hired drab; St. Francis of Assisi renouncing all for the sake of an unseen Christ — the moods of all these are at least one in this impulse away from self.

Incredulity concerning Dante's childish love for Beatrice is thus based on a misunderstanding of what Dante meant. How, it has often been asked, could a nine-year-old boy, in whom the sex-instinct is not yet developed, experience such a passion? There is no question of sexual passion. There was never any question of that, so far as we may trust his word, between Dante and Beatrice. But whoever denies that small boys may "love" little girls adoringly, devotedly, may perform miracles of juvenile self-sacrifice for their sakes, is a person of singularly limited experience and observation. Whatever, if any, psychological distinction there may be between such "puppy love," and childish love for father or mother or nurse, at least the impulse of self-devotion, common indeed to both, is observably stronger in the former. Dante's child-love then is perfectly normal; that it was the beginning of a religious conversion he only recognized long afterward.

When recognized, this spontaneous altruistic impulse in love became the basis of Dante's religious experience, and the motive of all his poetry. To feel and follow the impulse is to be

truly noble, to have a "*cor gentile*," a gentle heart.
To reveal it as the power within ourselves which
makes for blessedness is the mission of the "sweet
new style," the message which, as Dante says, —

> . . . in that manner
> Which love within me dictates, I go declaring.

Dante's poetry is the story of this impulse
implanted by love; of its growth from a casual
and passing mood into a master passion reaching
out, not to one other human being only, but to
all humanity, and from humanity, by the leading
of faith, to humanity's God. It is the saving
grace : those who have not felt it, and only those,
are damned. For all love, however base else,
however dark its desire, yet in this impulse, so
far looks to, leads to, the light. Therefore is
Beatrice able to say that the "eternal light"
shines through all love; and that,

> . . . if aught else lure your love,
> Naught is it save some vestige of that light,
> Ill understood, which there is shining through.
> *Paradiso*, v, 10–12.

Her assurance is no vagary of medieval mysticism,
no fallacy of a mind in vertigo, which as it spins
blurs the real variety of things into a confused
oneness; but a recognition of the observable

psychological fact that there is in all love, highest
and lowest, a stirring of generous emotion.

Precisely because the altruism of love is a spontaneous impulse, it is demonstrable only by experience, by involuntary experience. Only the
lover understands the lover; hence Dante is
continually declaring that he addresses those
only "that have intelligence of love." Nor is
he preaching love. The commandment, "Thou
shalt love thy neighbor," is unconstitutional to our
nature: we cannot love to order; we fall, not
jump, in love. Dante's teacher, St. Thomas
Aquinas, rightly distinguishes two psychological
moments in love, a *"passio"* and a *"virtus,"* an
impression which evokes an expression. Both
indeed are independent of our reason and will:
of the impression we are passively receptive; in
the expression our nature responds spontaneously,
if at all. It is strange that Francesca da Rimini
should plead to Dante for

Love, that exempts no one beloved from loving.

For did Dante himself find requital of his love
from the living Beatrice? or did he blame her for
her indifference to him? On the contrary, even
when she denied him her salutation, — that
which had been his "blessedness," and the mere
anticipation of which had kindled *"una fiamma di*

caritate," a glow of good-will towards all men, —
even then, far from complaining or long repining,
he came to find his still greater blessedness in the
pure altruism of love which gives all, asking nothing. In her will is his peace.

With this mood of self-renunciation begins, as
he himself tells, his true "new life," and "the
matter new and nobler" of the "sweet new style."
But although Dante is now withdrawn into himself, and asks no least response from his lady, his
mood is far from the bastard platonism of the
Renaissance, as pithily summarized, for instance,
in Michelangelo's quatrain : —

> Mentre ch' alla beltà ch' i' viddi in prima
>   Apresso l' alma, che per gli occhi vede,
>   L' immagin dentro crescie, e quella cede
> Quasi vilmente e senza alcuna stima.

Which may be roughly paraphrased : —

> While to the beauty which I first regarded
>   I turn my soul, that through mine eyes perceiveth,
>   Within my soul that beauty's image liveth,
> Itself as base and worthless is discarded.

Michelangelo means, of course, that, possessing
the idea of beauty abstracted from the particular
beautiful thing, — woman or other, — we have
no further use for the thing ; we are not concerned
to pull up after us the ladder we have climbed by.

But Dante did not discard Beatrice as a thing *"senza alcuna stima,"* nothing worth. He may have idealized the woman; but it was the woman still, though idealized, that inspired him. Her individual personality, her particular and unique beauty of body and soul, was for him the greatly precious thing in heaven as upon earth. She is for him no stepping-stone to higher things, which, having served its purpose, is left behind. His last word to her in heaven is a prayer to her as an immortal personality, close indeed to the Divine Personality, but not merged or lost in that. Platonic love, humanly speaking, is selfish: it envisages the one beloved as a provocative to its own contemplative raptures. There is something almost vampirish in this going about imaginatively sucking off the sweets of girls and things just to stock up one's own mental honeycomb. The very essence of Dante's love is its unselfishness. To mark the contrast after the manner of his own allegorical vision, it is not he that fed on Beatrice's beauty, it is she that fed on his heart, that absorbed his desire and will.

It does not appear that Dante ever asked or desired from Beatrice requital of his love; it does appear that he did desire and ask from other women requital of his passion. Boccaccio imputed to him an amatorious disposition; and there are those of his poems which bear out the imputation. He himself confessed and attempted to avoid scandal attaching to certain adventures. Those two ladies whom he professes to have used as "screens" to conceal his ideal love for Beatrice, doubtless did so — by being real loves; and that lady compassionate who consoled him a while after Beatrice's death probably turned his thought from heaven in a way not unheard of before or since. Beatrice's caustic rebuke on the summit of the Mount of Purgatory may well have been for other fallings-off also, — Dante's words almost always carry double, — but it invited most, I think, his last and most intimate purgation, by penitence, of the cardinal sin against the very principle of redemption, — pure and unselfish love. Yet the admission of these impure loves is no bar to belief in a pure love coexistent. Even a Paul Verlaine may profess in his *Sagesse* sincere adoration of the Virgin, along with profanest passion in his *Parallèlement.*

Within this earthly temple there's a crowd;

and some sanctify the temple as a house of prayer, and some make it a den of thieves.

The disinterestedness of Dante's love for Beatrice does not, however, reduce it to friendship or hero-worship. He felt the subtle appeal of sex also, but as an appeal for his consciousness translated wholly into terms of tenderness and self-devotion. Let me emphasize again the sanity of his mood over against the essential morbidness of most so-called "platonic love," or "courtly love," or "chivalric love." The motive common to these social and literary fashions, so widely current in the Middle Ages and Renaissance, is, broadly speaking, a desire to have your dance without paying the fiddler, to devise ways and means of playing with fire without getting burned. Philandering was never dreamed of in Plato's own philosophy; and the mood of philandering is almost always morbid, when it is not merely sensualism in masquerade. But Dante tells no tale of self-indulgence in luxurious emotional titillation, of *entretiens d'amour* — or "dam-foolishness." His homage is not that of obsequious vassal to capricious lord, but of the redeemed to the Saviour; for it was she that evoked in him the spirit of sacrifice which is the beginning of redemption.

In the *Divine Comedy*, indeed, it would at first sight seem that he at least imaginatively assumes requital of his love: the transfigured Beatrice condescends to him, lovingly uplifts him. "Love moved me," she tells her messenger, Virgil. Yet Dante, as he proceeds, shows clearly that moving love to be not personal, not the yearning of the individual soul to the individual soul, but a saintly charity, responsive by its nature to all, directed to him only because of his especial appeal to her in his need. Indeed, in her high place in heaven beside the ancient Rachel, she had even been oblivious of his need, until Lucia, sent by the Virgin herself, mother of charity, "meridian torch of charity," pleaded with her in his behalf. He is to her but her "friend," her "brother," in Christ. Or if a warmer impulse is awakened in her, it is that of motherhood, womanly spontaneous at the call of need : —

> . . . She after a pitying sigh,
> Her eyes directed towards me with that look
> A mother casts on a delirious child.
> *Paradiso*, i, 100–102 (Longfellow).

To her he turns as a little tired child to its mother : —

> Oppressed with stupor, I unto my guide
> Turned like a little child who always runs
> For refuge there where he confideth most ;
>
> And she, even as a mother who straightway
> Gives comfort to her pale and breathless boy
> With voice whose wont it is to reassure him,
>
> Said to me, etc.
> *Paradiso*, xxii, 1–7 (Longfellow).

Symbolic of their spiritual relationship is the aspect of their physical ascent: —

> Beatrice upward gazed, and I on her.
>
> *Paradiso*, ii, 22.

Very different from this almost hieratic condescension is Margaret's intimate gladness at Faust's redemption. Margaret sees her lover returned, not merely to goodness, to God, but to herself, for herself to love and cherish and serve in heaven as on earth, only more perfectly and forever. The *Mater Gloriosa* has not to plead for him with her; it is she who makes passionate appeal to the *Mater Gloriosa:* —

> Incline, O Maiden,
> With Mercy laden,
> In light unfading,
> Thy gracious countenance upon my bliss!
> My loved, my lover,
> His trials over
> In yonder world, returns to me in this! . . .
> Vouchsafe to me that I instruct him!
> Still dazzles him the Day's new glare.

And the Virgin advises her: —

> Rise, then, to higher spheres! Conduct him,
> Who feeling thee, shall follow there!
>
> *Faust*, Part ii, Act v, Scene 7 (Taylor).

In those higher spheres, Faust is presumably to be reunited forever with Margaret. Not so may

Dante hope. Once her saving mission accomplished, Beatrice also rises to her own higher sphere, where she is forthwith, Dante once more forgotten, rapt in contemplation wholly of God.

> . . . She, so far away,
> Smiled, as it seemed, and looked once more at me;
> Then unto the eternal fountain turned.
>> *Paradiso*, xxxi, 91–93 (Longfellow).

Beatrice in heaven, then, remains for him what she had been on earth — a mover of personal love, herself unmoved by personal love. The same spirit of *caritate*, of loving-kindness, with which he, enamored, identified her, living, is the principle of his apotheosis of her, dead. The real Beatrice may have merited the apotheosis, may have been such an incarnation of loving-kindness, or not — who can say? Dante, loving her, thought so, — even as every Jack in love thinks his Jill. The illusion is primal. But the only tragedy of illusion is disillusionment; and in the chance for disillusionment is the risk of requited love. For that blessedness in renunciation which Dante declared "cannot grow less," there is also a cynical justification: who renounces union with one beloved assures himself against that contempt which familiarity may — though of course need not — breed. Indeed, if Dante himself was altogether innocent of the cynicism, he must have been singular in his time. The time held woman the inferior animal, to whom man must rationally condescend, could not rationally look up. It soberly believed, as Leopardi later, that

> . . . that which is in gentle hearts inspired
> By her own beauty, woman dreams not of,
> Nor yet might understand.

There may be serious question, therefore, if Dante's religious experience of love could for him have remained religious had Beatrice proved kind. A Lovelace in a modern French play, being informed by his married mistress that, suddenly widowed, she is now ready to marry him, exclaims in consternation, "*Mais, madame, je vous aime en homme du monde!*" One feels, not intending irreverence, that Dante must have answered Beatrice, yielding, "*Mais, madame, je vous aime en homme d'autremonde!*" Tennyson's idealization in *The Princess* of love in domesticity, love in harness pulling toward a common goal of ideal good, was hardly thinkable for Dante. The reason was not, I think, that the code of "chivalric love," by Andreas Capellanus, redactor of the code, had declared "*amorem non posse inter duos jugales suas extendere vires,*" love to be incapable of extending its power over the wedded.

Dante never bowed to code or dogma — even
highest dogma of the Church — without question ;
for him ever

> . . . springs up, in fashion of a shoot,
> Doubt at the foot of truth.
>
> *Paradiso*, iv, 130, 131 (Longfellow).

For him, behind the code must appear the sanction ; and at least one sanction of Andreas's code
was experience.   As a fact of experience, marriage
in the Middle Ages was not of a nature to justify
Tennyson's idealization.   There may be question
if marriage is altogether commonly so yet.

In one sense, then, the inaccessibility, the
"splendid isolation," of Beatrice was a fortunate
accident.   Because of it, Dante's religious experience of love was saved from possible disillusionment.   Experiencing the instinctive altruism of
love, he was able, uninhibited, to project the color
of his own mood into her nature who had evoked
his mood.   For Dante explicitly concedes nobleness of impulse to woman, while he denies to her
reasoned and seasoned virtue.   In his ode on true
nobility, he declares, —

> Gentlehood is wherever there is virtue,
> But virtue not wherever gentlehood ;
> Even as the heaven is wherever is the star.
> But not the converse holds.

> And we in women and in youthful age
> Discern this saving grace,
> So far as they are held to be shamefast,
> Which yet's not virtue, —

but is — as he explains in his commentary on the ode — "*certa passion buona,*" an estimable emotion. Such in Beatrice was that *caritate,* unreflective, passional, the essence of her womanliness, her spiritual beauty. Awakened by her in him, the emotion becomes through his masculine reflection self-conscious, understood; and so is translated from an instinctive emotion to a rational virtue. This virtue his reason recognizes as identical in principle with "*la prima virtù,*" the supreme virtue of God, —

> The love that moves the sun and other stars.

In this sense. Beatrice the woman is for Dante the symbol of the lovable God. She is no mere allegory, in which truth is infolded "in covert veil" by the poet's own ingenuity. She has religious significance as a symbol, precisely as the Communion when the "Real Presence" is admitted: God lovable is "truly, really, and substantially" contained in her, as after the consecration of the bread and wine, Christ is "truly, really, and substantially contained under the species of those sensible things." Hence the

symbolism of the *New Life* — the association of
Beatrice with the mystic number nine, "of which
the root is the Blessed Trinity;" the esoteric
significance of her name, as "Blessedness;" the
daring intimation of her identity with the Christ
Himself — this symbolism is not poetic fantasy or
amorous hyperbole, but spiritual truth. In her
presence he is as in the presence of God; and therefore his own visions and tremblings and swoonings
and exaltations, morbid or incredible in a mere
human lover, are normal and familiar in the religious convert of all ages.

Dante's was a time of peculiar religious sensibility; but turning instead to the matter-of-fact
nineteenth century and the prosaic United States,
consider the conversion, the "new life," of the young
Methodist Bradley, cited by William James in his
Varieties of Religious Experience. The confession of
the obscure young American throws a strange backward light on that of the great Florentine poet.
"At first," Bradley says, "I began to feel my
heart beat very quick all on a sudden, which made
me at first think that perhaps something is going
to ail me, though I was not alarmed, for I felt no
pain. My heart increased in its beating, which
soon convinced me that it was the Holy Spirit
from the effect it had on me." So at first sight
of Beatrice, Dante's heart beat *"fortemente,"*

and he recognized the coming of the "*deus fortior me*," — which was divine love, even as the Holy Spirit is love.

Bradley continues: "I began to feel exceedingly happy and humble, and such a sense of unworthiness as I had never felt before. I could not very well help speaking out, which I did, and said, Lord, I do not deserve this happiness, or words to that effect, while there was a stream (resembling air in feeling) came into my mouth and heart in a more sensible manner than that of drinking anything, which continued, as near as I could judge, five minutes or more, which appeared to be the cause of such a palpitation of my heart. It took complete possession of my soul, and I am certain that I desired the Lord, while in the midst of it, not to give me any more happiness, for it seemed as if I could not contain what I had got. My heart seemed as if it would burst, but it did not stop until I felt as if I was unutterably full of the love and grace of God . . . and all the time that my heart was a-beating, it made me groan like a person in distress, which was not very easy to stop, though I was in no pain at all."

Compare with this singular ecstasy Dante's declaration, in the eleventh chapter of the *New Life*, of the effects upon himself of Beatrice's salutation: how a flame of charity possessed him

which made him pardon whosoever had offended
him ; how he could answer any one who spoke to
him only "love !" with a countenance clothed in
humility ; how when she actually saluted him,
at the unbearable beatitude, his body many times
fell like a heavy lifeless thing. The similarity of
emotional experience is obvious.

Even Dante's proneness to visions and to inter-
course with spiritual presences finds its counter-
part in Bradley : "And while I lay reflecting, after
my heart stopped beating, feeling as if my soul
was full of the Holy Spirit, I thought that perhaps
there might be angels hovering round my bed.   I
felt just as if I wanted to converse with them, and
finally I spoke, saying, 'O ye affectionate angels !
how is it that ye can take so much interest in our
welfare, and we take so little interest in our own ?'"

And lastly, the resulting mood for Bradley, as
for Dante, was a passionate desire for release from
self, and an expansive impulse of altruism.   In
the morning, continues Bradley, "I got up to dress
myself, and found to my surprise that I could but
just stand.   It appeared to me as if it was a little
heaven upon earth.   My soul felt as completely
raised above the fears of death as of going to
sleep ; and like a bird in a cage, I had a desire,
if it was the will of God, to get release from my
body and to dwell with Christ, though willing to

E

do good to others, and to warn sinners to repent."
So saying, he but says more crudely : —

> . . . Already my desire and will were turned —
> Even as a wheel revolving evenly —
> By the Love that moves the sun and other stars.

I have dwelt on this curious analogy, because it
seems to me to refute the contention that the
extremes of sensibility in the *New Life* are to be
taken as mere amorous and literary convention.
Of course, Dante employed the parlance of his
masters in love-poetry, just as he must, drawing
an angel, have produced a figure which we should
call Giottesque. A conventionalized phraseology does not imply necessarily an unoriginal
thought any more than a conventionalized frock-
coat implies necessarily an unoriginal man. Orig-
inality is not the same thing as eccentricity.
The "sweet new style" was, in the first instance,
simply the old garment covering a new man ; as
the man grew and expanded, doubtless the garment was little by little altered to fit.

In the *New Life* Beatrice is the symbol of the
lovable God ; in the *Divine Comedy*, she is still
this, and more. She is the symbol of God's
omniscience as well. To love her had been to
love God ; now to know her is to know God.
Again, she is no mere allegory of theology, no

personified abstraction like the innumerable didactic phantoms — "Lady Meed" or "Dame
Sapience" or "Sister Rightwiseness" — of medieval evocation. With the woman's body she
has put off the woman's limitations. Illuminated
by the divine reason, her passive goodness has
developed into active virtue, *knowing* the good
which it desires and wills. Therefore at the last,
Dante is justified in saying to her in heaven what
he would have thought it fantastic to say to any
woman on earth : —

> Of whatsoever things I have beheld
>   I recognize the grace and potency,
> Even through thy power and thine excellence.
> *Paradiso*, xxxi, 82–84.

Of course, as need hardly be said, Dante is here
imaginatively projecting his own illuminated
intelligence into the mind of his immortal lady, as
in the *New Life* he had projected his mood of
charity into her mortal heart. It was in each case
an act of loving faith. If she really lived here on
earth, she may have been what he believed her
to be. In any case, the burden of disproof, both
of her existence and of her excellence, is upon him
who doubts. At present, there is no evidence
against, and there is some evidence for, her being
Bice Fortinari, a real Florentine girl and woman.

I cannot but hope that the present interpretation of Dante's love for her may relieve their possible relations of any seeming unnaturalness, and at the same time explain how it came to pass that this love grew for him into a religious experience, leading him to conversion and confidence of ultimate redemption.

Experience of the spontaneous altruism of love, — this alone is the major premise of his whole syllogism of life. It is in all love : neither Dante nor, for that matter, Goethe asserts that only the "woman-love" leads us upward. But as sex-love is the most intense love that mankind at large normally experiences, it is most, or only, in sex-love that the still, small voice of *caritate*, of self-devotion, is heard. Finally, therefore, it is as the supreme expression of this religious experience, in a phase at once most universal and most intense, that Dante's poetry is a "criticism of life," not medieval life, but human life.

THE ORACLE OF LOVE IN THE TWELFTH CHAPTER OF "LA VITA NUOVA"

I

AFTER Beatrice had denied to him her salutation, Dante declares that Love appeared to him in a vision, and sighed, and said: "*Fili mi, tempus est ut prætermittantur simulacra nostra —* my son, it is time for us to lay aside our counterfeiting;" and that, having so said, Love wept for pity, and to Dante, asking, "Lord of nobleness, why dost thou weep?" replied: "*Ego tamquam centrum circuli, cui simili modo se habent circumferentiæ partes; tu autem non sic —* I am as the centre of a circle, for which all parts of the circumference are alike; but thou art not so." Perplexed, Dante again asked: "What thing is this, Master, that thou hast spoken thus darkly?" Love only replied: "Demand no more than may be useful to thee."

Love's injunction, "it is time for us to lay aside our counterfeiting," is clear. Beatrice, and others,

had misunderstood Dante's "screening" homage
to another lady; it is time, therefore, to confess
the truth to his real lady. Obediently, Dante
addresses to Beatrice a *ballata*, which says of its
maker: —

> Lady his heart has been
> of such fixed constancy
> that his each thought incites him to serve thee:
> early 'twas thine, and never hath it strayed.

Apparently, this obedience, though due, is to
entail disaster for Dante, because he is not, like
Love, "as the centre of a circle, for which all parts
of the circumference are alike." Also, present
understanding of what Love means would not
avail to avert the disaster, otherwise an explanation would be "useful." We should expect,
accordingly, to find the key to the oracular utterance in the direct consequences of Dante's obedi-
ent "laying aside of counterfeiting."

After this above written vision [Dante writes], when
I had already said those words [to Beatrice] which Love
had charged me to say, many and divers thoughts
began to assail and tempt me, each one almost irresistibly, among which thoughts four seemed most to
disturb my life's repose. The first whereof was this:
The lordship of Love is good since it draweth the mind
of his liege from all evil things. The next was this:
The lordship of Love is not good since the more faith
his liege beareth him, the more heavy and more grievous

straits must he pass.   The next was this: The name
of Love is so sweet to hear that it seemeth to me impossible that its action in most things be other than
sweet. . . .   The fourth was this: The lady for whom
Love constraineth thee thus is not as other ladies that
her heart be lightly moved.   And each assailed me
so, that it made me stand like one who knoweth not
by which path to take his way, and who fain would
go, yet knoweth not whither to turn.   And if I thought
that I would seek a way common to all, namely, where
all might be in accord, this way was most inimical to
me, namely, to call upon and yield me to the arms of
pity.

Drawn "irresistibly" four ways in turn, Dante
is obviously in a position unlike "the centre of a
circle, for which all parts of the circumference are
alike."   Concerned as he is for his own welfare,
he can see no way out, no center of accord, except
in his lady's pity, which he forebodes must be
"inimical."

The foreboding is immediately justified.   From
Beatrice he finds not pity, but mockery.   So far
from pity making accord between his four conflicting thoughts, his appeal to pity only involved
him in a new fourfold mystery —

whereof the first [matter] is, that ofttimes I grieved
when memory moved my fancy to imagine how Love
dealt with me.   The second is how Love did many
times suddenly assail me so mightily that there remained
naught in me of life save a thought that spake of this

lady; the third is, that when this battle of love assailed me thus, I set forth, as 'twere all pallid, to behold this lady, believing that the sight of her would defend me from this assault, forgetting what befel me through drawing nigh to such gentleness; the fourth is, how that such sight not only did not defend me, but finally discomfited the small remnant of my life.

Thus the lover seems at the point of spiritual death, when suddenly all is changed. Dante presently announces "a new matter and more noble than the past." Questioned as to the end of his love, he replies: "Ladies mine, the end of my love was once this lady's salutation. . . . But since it hath pleased her to deny it to me, Love, my lord, by his grace hath placed all my beatitude in that which cannot fail me," namely, as he says presently, "in those words which praise my lady."

Love, "lord of nobleness," has at last revealed himself to Dante, whose own love to now has been ignoble, because self-centered, craving reward in the salutation. The four thoughts which drew him from his repose were all for his own welfare. Henceforth his love is to be centered in self-effacing service, in pure homage. He will give all, asking nothing; and therefore he can lose nothing. Not pity, his "enemy" indeed, but renunciation, was signified by that "center of indifference" to which Love, "lord of nobleness,"

had likened himself. Such love Dante joyously
believes he has now found, and declares in the
sonnet, "Love and the gentle heart are but one
thing." In the canzone, "Ladies that have
intelligence of love," he first expresses this "new
matter and nobler" of love, this selfless homage.
It is significant that Bonagiunta cites (*Purgatorio*,
xxiv, 51) this canzone as demarking the "sweet
new style," when asking Dante to define that
style. To him Dante replies: —

> I am one who, when
> Love me inspireth, note, and in such wise
> as he dictates within, go setting forth.

The "oracle of Love" in the twelfth chapter
of the *Vita Nuova* is just such a dictation.
Love's obscurely declared nature, when realized
by Dante through mistake and suffering, is what
turns Dante's "young life" into his "new life,"
his regenerate life, when his selfish love is born
again in the new intelligence of the love which is
nobleness.

But fulfillment of love through self-renunciation
is not yet perfect. While Beatrice lives, Dante has
at least the reward of her presence. Presently,
death robs him of even that. He despairs, and
turns for comfort to the Pitiful Lady (*la donna
pietosa*). Again forgetful of the nemesis which

appeal to pity brought, again misunderstanding
the love which is nobleness, he said within himself :
"It cannot be but that noble love is with that
pitiful lady." And he thought of her : "This is
a gentle lady, fair, young, and wise, and hath appeared perchance by Love's will, in order that my
life may find rest." But such was not the will
of Love, "lord of nobleness." His life does not
find rest, but is distracted by a new "battle of
thoughts," by one justifying selfish solace, another
commanding unselfish loyalty. For a while the
selfish thought dominates, until "a mighty
vision" of young Beatrice leaves him penitent,
and filled with "tribulation" such that his eyes
weep so

> that Love
> encircleth them as with a martyr's crown.

Thus this spiritual crisis recorded in the fortieth
chapter exactly repeats that already recorded in
the sixteenth. In each case, centering his love in
pity, he is at once drawn opposite ways by contrary thoughts, and is then suddenly confronted
with Beatrice, first in the flesh, the second time
in "a mighty vision" (una forte immaginazione).
On the one occasion her girlish mockery, on the
other the silent reproach of the girlish figure he
had first seen and loved, utterly discomfits him.

From each discomfiture springs the realization
that the true "center" of the love which is nobleness lies not in the solace of indulgent pity, but
in the self-devotion of the "gentle heart." The
ignoble lover seeks to realize his own self-will, and
finds only unrest and despair; the noble lover
submits his own will to the will of his beloved.
After the first crisis, Love, by his grace, had taught
Dante the unfailing beatitude of selfless contemplation and praise of his lady mortal; so now, after
the second crisis, Love will teach the still higher
beatitude of praise and ideal contemplation of
her immortal. In the last sonnet of the *Vita
Nuova* this "new intelligence" is dictated by
Love. Drawn ever upwards by a "new intelligence that Love, weeping, implants in it," his
"pilgrim spirit" soars to the Empyrean, where it
beholds Beatrice in glory, yet is incapable of
rightly declaring that glory.

Love, dictating this new intelligence of himself,
weeps — as he had wept when first, after the denial of the salutation, he had declared darkly his
true nature. Evidently not even yet is Dante's
love fully subdued to the love which is nobleness.
Before his "pilgrim spirit" may fully realize and
declare the glory of Beatrice, that is of Love himself (the identity had been revealed by Love in
chapter twenty-four), it must pass through Hell

and Purgatory; must again, after its errancy, be
confronted with Beatrice, and, appealing to pity,
seem to find pity an "enemy" still. Though
angels are moved to pity by his misery, Beatrice is
sternly unrelenting. In his manhood, as in his
"young life," he must pay the "scot that sheddeth
tears." At Beatrice's rebuke, —

Then at my heart there gnawed so great remorse that
I fell stricken (*Paradiso*, xxxi, 88–89).

But after this third and last crisis, Love finally
reveals himself fully in the knowledge of his kingdom, Paradise. Drawn upward to the Empyrean
again, as his "pilgrim spirit" had been drawn in
the *Vita Nuova*, Dante now sees not only Beatrice in her glory, but the Godhead also — this
last as "three circles of threefold color, and of one
dimension," of which the third seemed to be "fire
that was breathed forth equally by both" the
other two. This third circle symbolizes the power
of the Holy Ghost, or Love. Dante's mortal
faculties failed to sustain the beatific vision; but
not until already his

> desire and will were rolled,
> even as a wheel that evenly is moved,[1]
> by the Love that moves the sun and other stars.

[1] The word "evenly" or "equally" (*egualmente*), applied
to the moving wheel, itself implies the same idea as is contained
in Love's self-description: both the wheel to which Dante

That is to say, having at last realized the Divine
Circle, the one ray, the virtual center of which is
Love, Dante's whole moral nature is subdued to
harmony with that Love, and becomes *concentric*
with it.   Selfish desire and self-will are quenched;
he is able to say with the blessed, in Piccarda's
words: —

In His will is our peace.

Now Beatrice's seemingly "inimical" denial
of pity is explained.   In the *Vita Nuova* (chap.
xxiv) Dante had foreshadowed her relation to
him as that of Christ to the sinner.   "Whom the
Lord loveth he chasteneth;"   it was Beatrice's
chastening which at last made Dante's love also
"as the center of a circle, for which all parts of
the circumference are alike" — that is to say, as
we may now interpret, not a selfish passion blown
hither and thither by the four winds of desire,
but a joyous acquiescence in the will of the loved
one, a "center of indifference," such as Piccarda
intends when she answers Dante (*Paradiso*, iii,
70–72) : —

Brother, the quality of perfect love (*carità*)
stilleth our will, and maketh us desire
but what we have, nor giveth other thirst.

compares himself regenerate, and the circle of which Love
declares himself the center, are true circles; there is no un-
evenness, no inequality, in the circumference (*simili modo se
habent circumferentiæ partes — ad centrum*).

But while seeking nothing for itself, this perfect love is a radiant center of loving charity equally for all. In heaven, where all are such radiant centers of love, there is, indeed, no distinction between giving and receiving; all are as "centers of circles, for which all parts of the circumference are alike," since, as Virgil says (*Purgatorio,* xv, 73–75) : —

> The more on high who one another know,
> the more are to love well, the more love is,
> and like a mirror each to each gives back.

As if to symbolize visually Love's self-description, Dante represents the spirits of the more blessed as literally centers of flaming circles. The spirits in the Moon appear as merely shadowy human forms; in Mercury the shadowy forms begin to glow; in the higher planets the glow hides the inclosed form, and the spirit voices sound from the centers of these "torches" or "suns" or "splendors." One spirit, San Pier Damiano, is explicitly described as "love" at the center of a whirling circle of light (*Paradiso*, xxi, 79 ff.) ; and the Virgin Mary becomes the center of "a radiance circle-formed around her," by "the angelic love" of Raphael (*Paradiso*, xxiii, 94 ff.). Finally the Godhead appears as a threefold circle, within which Dante seems to see the image of Christ, that is to say, of Love himself. Visually regarded, Love's dark words in the *Vita Nuova* could not be more fully justified.

If the above interpretation of these dark words be correct, they are by no means the mere *obiter dictum* or even unexplained mystification that the commentators have left them, but form the dramatic announcement, and contain the essential tenet, of the religion of love embodied in the "sweet, new style" of both the *Vita Nuova* and the *Divina Commedia*.

II

This symbolizing of moral perfection by the geometric "equality" of a circle, and comparison of the love "which is nobleness" to the center of a circle, is anticipated by St. Augustine in his dialogue entitled *De quantitate animæ*.[1] To illustrate how the incorporeal soul may exert power even over the material body, Augustine has recourse to pure mathematics. By a series of Socratic questions, he brings his young interlocutor, Evodius, to agree that of all plane figures the circle is the most perfect in "equality," in that its circumference is everywhere equivalent (*concors*),

---

[1] *Patrologiæ Latinæ*, Tom. xxxii, 1035 *et seq.* Dante himself cites the dialogue in the epistle to Can Grande, sec. 28.

its "equality" is broken by no angle, and from its center to all parts of the circumference equal lines can be drawn (*et a cujus medio ad omnes extremitatis partes pares liniæ duci possunt*). We are reminded at once of Love's words to Dante.

But why Evodius's instinctive preference for such geometrical "equality," or symmetry? Really, explains his mentor, the instinct is at bottom the recognition of "high and inviolable justice." Justice is based on equity; equity is so called from equality. Thus the circle is a *natural* symbol of justice.

The determinant and measure of a circle, however, is the mathematical point, its center. For a circle is described by the revolution of the point at the end of the radial line about the fixed point at the other end. And by definition, a mathematical point, having neither length, breadth, or thickness, is incorporeal. In potency and incorporeality, therefore, it is a natural symbol of the soul; and, when the moving center of a circle, a natural symbol of the just soul, that is, of a soul "conforming equally on all sides to reason."

Certainly, Augustine's explanation exactly fits the self-definition of Dante's Love, "lord of nobleness," or virtue. Virtue for Dante, as for Augustine, is "a certain divine harmony of relations" (*divina quadam congruentia rationum*) in the soul.

Love denies to Dante present possession of this "divine harmony" of soul : hence the tribulations which follow in the *Vita Nuova*.   A later passage in Augustine's treatise helps to motivate these tribulations.

In this passage Augustine traces in neo-platonic fashion the seven grades of ascent of the human soul back to God.   In the first, or lowest, grade, the soul is life-force without consciousness, that which we have in common with the plants ; in the second grade, it is sentient, but not rational, that which we have in common with the brutes ; in the third grade it is rational, but not moral. The wisdom of this third grade is worldly wisdom. With the fourth grade, divine wisdom enters in to purge the soul of worldliness and selfishness ; in the fifth grade, the purged soul confirms itself in its "new life" by works of piety and charity ; in the sixth grade, it yearns in contemplation from afar for that blessedness of union with God, which is its Sabbath, or seventh grade.   But no grade in this ascent, no rung in this ladder of love, may with impunity be skipped ; there are no short cuts to blessedness.   The highest good is indeed to behold God ; but "whosoever would do this before they are cleansed and healed, are so stricken by that light of truth that they see in it not only no goodness, but even much evil,

F

and therefore deny to it the name of truth, and
with their lusts and miserable pleasures, refusing
health, flee away in their darkness, which is even
their death." So Dante, yearning for the reward
of Beatrice (blessedness) before he is healed and
cleansed, is tempted to call love an evil thing, to flee
from Beatrice, from blessedness itself, because it
chastens; and he is racked by conflicting im-
pulses, until he feels his death at hand. He is
saved by turning his over-presumptuous soul
back to the neglected fourth grade of self-purga-
tion, finding his peace in selfless worship. Only
will he be worthy of the reward (*mercede*) of
Beatrice, or blessedness, when his love shall have
become also as the center of a circle that is moved,
like a wheel *equally*,

By the love which moves the sun and the other stars.

THE PHILOSOPHY OF LOVE OF
GUIDO CAVALCANTI

In 1283 the young Dante sent out among the best-known Italian poets a sonnet asking interpretation of a dream. The god of love, so it seemed, had come carrying Beatrice asleep, and had fed her with Dante's own heart, and had then departed weeping.

Several poets answered. One, Dante of Maiano, suggested as a probable solution of this, and other such distressing visions, a dose of salts; the others fell in with Dante's mood and answered seriously. Of their various interpretations that which best pleased Dante, though not quite satisfied him, was Guido Cavalcanti's. "And this," wrote Dante later in the *New Life*, "was, as it were, the beginning of the friendship between him and me, when he knew that I was he who had sent it (the sonnet) to him."

Guido's interpretation was in an important particular ambiguous. Love, he wrote, fed your heart to your lady, seeing that "*vostra donna la morte chedea.*" To understand this clause as

67

meaning "Death claimed your lady" is natural,
and would make the interpretation interestingly
prophetic; but, whether or not this reading might
be justified symbolically, Dante himself forbids
it. For, in spite of his pleasure in his "first
friend's" explanation of the dream, he added:
"The true meaning of this dream was not then
seen by any one, but now it is plain to the sim-
plest." It was easy for him after the event to
read prophecy of Beatrice's death into the dream;
but he expressly denies to Guido among the rest
the prescience. We are bound, therefore, to take
as the interpreter's meaning that there was malice
prepense in the cannibal appetite of the sleeping
lady, that she claimed the death of her servant's
heart. No wonder the love god wept as he carried her off sated!

Irreverent though it be, one thinks of *The
Vampire* of Kipling. For Guido the gentle
Beatrice was as "the woman who couldn't understand," sucking, asleep, in a sort of diabolical
innocence, the life blood, literally eating the
heart, out of her helpless victim. And Dante,
the lover, the victim, approves the picture!

Of course the gruesomeness of this symbolism
may be explained away as merely a conceitfully
emphatic reassertion of the ancient fancy that a
lover's heart is no longer his own, but has passed

into the custody of his mistress.   Only, the dream
then and its interpretation would indeed be a
much ado about nothing.   And why, at so cus-
tomary a happening, should love weep?   In fact,
Guido's thought cuts deeper, and is, I venture
to urge, not so remote, in a sense, from the thought
underlying *The Vampire*.   It is *The Vampire*
uplifted into the more tenuous, yet no less intense,
atmosphere of mysticism.

Before attempting to let in light directly upon
this dim utterance it is expedient to recall certain
facts in Guido's life and personality.

"Cortese e ardito, ma sdegnoso e solitario e
intento allo studio" — so Guido is introduced into
the *Florentine Chronicle* of Dino Compagni, who
knew him personally.   Guido could not have been
much over twenty-five when, at the death of his
father, his elder brother being in orders, he became
head and champion of one of the two or three most
powerful and aristocratic families in the republic.
For generations the Cavalcanti had been leaders
in the state, haughtily contemptuous of the mere
people, yet fierce partisans of civic independence
against those who were willing to sacrifice this for
the dream of a "Greater Italy" united under a
revivified Emperor of the West.   To this great
feud and to the lesser local feuds which grew out of
it Guido may be said to have been a predestined,

yet mostly a willing, sacrifice. He was born into
the feud; he lived his life long in the heat of it;
it won him his wife; it perhaps lost him his best
friend; it certainly killed him before his time.

It won him his wife. In 1267, a year after the
decisive battle of Benevento, when the last hope
of the Imperialists, the Ghibellines, fell with
Manfred, an attempt in Florence was made toward
permanent peace by marrying together certain
sons and daughters of victors and vanquished.
Among the rest Guido Cavalcanti was wedded, or
then more likely betrothed, — for he could not
have been more than fifteen, — to Bice, daughter
of the Ghibelline leader, the Florentine "Corio-
lanus," Farinata degli Uberti. Seven years before
Farinata had "painted the Arbia red" with the
blood of Florentine Guelphs at Monteaperti;
and it had been a kinsman of Guido who commanded the Guelphs on that disastrous day. We
do not know how this real "Capulet-Montague"
match turned out, — only that Monna Bice bore
children to her husband and outlived him many
years, and that the peace which their union,
among others, was intended to effect did not
come to pass.

On the contrary the great Guelph families, after
1267 in secure possession of the city, soon quarreled,
even connived against each other with the ever

ready Ghibelline exiles, or with popular dema-
gogues, so great was their common jealousy.
Meanwhile, during the distraction of the nobles,
the middle classes had been prospering; and
coming at last to feel their strength and the
weakness of those above them, in 1293 they re-
belled and crushed the aristocrats. In the first
insolence of triumph they excluded the nobles
absolutely from public office, but two years later
conceded eligibility to such nobles as would join
one of the *Arti*, or trades-unions. This virtual
abdication of caste Guido Cavalcanti refused to
make. In vain good easy Dino pleaded with
him. "I am ever singing your praises," he wrote
in a kindly sonnet, "telling folks how wise you are,
and brave and strong, skilled to wield and ward
the sword, and how compact with sifted learning
your mind is, and how you can run and leap and
outlast the best. Nor is there lacking you high
birth nor wealth . . . in fine, the one thing
wanting to give scope to all these gifts and powers
is a mere name.

Ahi! com saresti stato om mercadiere!

Now almost certainly some generations back
the Cavalcanti had been in trade, and had made
their fortune in trade, but latterly it had pleased
them to entertain a genealogy reaching royally

back into Germany and descending into Italy with Charlemagne's baronage. To traverse this pleasing legend with the gross title "om merca-diere," tradesman, was out of the question: Guido declared himself irreconcilable.

Meanwhile Dante, unfettered by a legend or a temperament, had accepted the situation even cordially, and was taking active part in the councils of the new bourgeois régime. That Guido must have regarded his friend's secession with disgust seems natural. It was worse than an offense against party; it was an offense against caste. "Uomo vertudioso in molte cose, se non ch' egli era troppo tenero e stizzozo," writes Giovanni Villani of Guido. Fastidious, exclusive, thin-skinned, choleric, Guido was just the man to feel this consorting of his friend with vulgar political upstarts incompatible with their own intimacy. And the matter was made worse by its open denial of their poetic profession of faith in the "cor gentile." This vulgar folk was that "fango," that human "mud" of which Guinizelli had written: —

> Fere lo sole il fango tutto 'l giorno,
> Vile riman . . .

how might the "gentle heart" mix itself with this irredeemable "mud" and be not defiled? So

Guido addressed to his friend a sonnet at once haughty and tender — like Guido himself : [1] —

> Io vengo il giorno a te infinite volte
>   e trovoti pensar troppo vilmente :
>   allor mi dol de la gentil tua mente
>   e d'assai tue virtù che ti son tolte.
>
> Solevanti spiacer persone molte,
>   tuttor fuggivi la noiosa gente,
>   di me parlavi sì coralemente
>   che tutte le tue rime avei ricolte.
>
> Or non ardisco per la vil tua vita,
>   far mostramento che tu' dir mi piaccia,
>   nè vengo 'n guisa a te che tu mi veggi.
>
> Se 'l presente sonetto spesso leggi
>   lo spirito noioso che ti caccia
>   si partirà da l'anima invilita.[2]

[1] I believe that E. Lamma, in his *Questioni Dantesche*, Bologna, 1902, was the first to propose this construction of the famous "reproach." It seems to me the best of all.

> I come to thee infinite times a day
>   And find thee thinking too unworthily :
>   Then for thy gentle mind it grieveth me,
>   And for thy talents all thus thrown away.
>
> To flee the vulgar herd was once thy way,
>   To bar the many from thine amity ;
>   Of me thou spakest then full cordially
>   When thou hadst set thy verse in right array.
>
> But now I dare not, so thy life is base,
>   Make manifest that I approve thine art,
>   Nor come to thee so thou mayst see my face.
>
> Yet if this sonnet thou wilt take to heart,
>   The perverse spirit leading thee this chase
>   Out of thy soul polluted shall depart.

Whether the two friends again came together in life is not known. The next situation in which we hear of them is tragic. Dante is sitting among his "first friend's" judges; Guido is condemned to exile, and goes — in effect — to his death.

Under the new bourgeois rule civic disorders rather increased than otherwise. Prime mover of discord was the Florentine "Catiline," as Dino calls him, Corso Donati. Somewhat ineffectually opposing his self-seeking machinations were the *parvenu* Cerchi, powerful only through wealth and the popularity of their cause. With these also stood Guido. Hatred, no less than misfortune, makes strange bedfellows; and the hatred between Guido and Corso was intense. Each had sought the other's life; Corso meanly, by hired assassins; Guido openly, in the public street, by his own hand. Violence followed violence; the number of factionaries increased, until at last in 1300 the city Priors determined to expel the leaders of both parties. Guido was conspicuous among these leaders; Dante, as has been said, among these Priors. The place of exile, Sarzana, proved to be pestilent with fever; and although Guido and the Cerchi, less culpable than Corso, were recalled within the year, it was too late. A few months afterward, the 28th or

29th of August, 1300, Guido died. "*E fu gran dommaggio*," wrote Dino.

It was a strange preparation for "gentle and gracious rhymes of love," — this short, tumultuous, hate-driven career. Yet there is but one direct echo of the feudist in all Guido's verse, — a sonnet to a kinsman, Nerone Cavalcanti. Nerone had made Florence too hot for the rival Buondelmonti, and Guido hails him with ironical deprecation.

> Novelle ti so dire, odi, Nerone,
>   che' Bondelmonti treman di paura,
>   e tutt' i fiorentin' no li assicura,
>   udendo dir che tu a' cor di leone.
>
> E più treman di te che d'un dragone
>   veggendo la tua faccia, ch' è sì dura
>   che no la riterria ponte nè mura
>   se non la tomba del re faraone.
>
> De! com' tu fai grandissimo peccato
>   sì alto sangue voler discacciare,
>   chè tutti vanno via sanza ritegno.
>
> Ma ben è ver che ti largar lo pegno,
>   di che potrai l' anima salvare
>   se fossi paziente del mercato.[1]

[1] News have I for thee, Nero, in thine ear.
   They of the Buondelmonte quake with dread,
   Nor by all Florence may be comforted,
   For that thou hast a lion's heart they hear.

Guido's disdainful temper both piqued and puzzled his townsfolk. Sacchetti's anecdote [1] of the Florentine small boy who, having slyly nailed Guido's gown to his bench, then teased him until the irate gentleman tried — naturally to his discomfiture — to chase him, has its point in a very human satisfaction at the scorner scorned. Boccaccio's novella [2] is more significant, illustrating vividly, if perhaps by a fictitious occurrence only, the subtle mingling of awe and defiance which Guido inspired. Boccaccio's "character" of Guido is a eulogy. "He was one of the best thinkers (*loici*) in the world and an accomplished lay philosopher (*filosofo*

> And more than any dragon thee they fear,
> > For looking on thy face they are as dead:
> > Bastion nor bridge against it stands in stead,
> > Nor less than Pharaoh's grave were barrier.
>
> Marry! but thou hast done a wicked thing,
> > Having the heart to scatter such blue blood,
> > For without let now one and all they flee.
>
> And 'sooth, a truce-bait too they proffered thee,
> > So that thy soul might still be with the Good,
> > Hadst but had stomach for the bargaining.

For the first quatrain of this sonnet I have slightly altered Rossetti's translation. In the rest a mistaken understanding of the sonnet as if addressed to the pope has misled him.

[1] *Novella*, 68.
[2] *Decameron*, vi, 9.

naturale), . . . and withal a most engaging,
elegant, and affable gentleman, easily first in
whatever he undertook, and in all that befitted
his rank." This character, together with the
mood of tragic doubt upon which the point of
Boccaccio's narrative turns, inevitably, if tritely,
brings to mind Ophelia's character of Hamlet: —

The courtier's, soldier's, scholar's eye, tongue, sword;
The expectancy and rose of the fair state,
The glass of fashion and the mould of form,
The observed of all observers. . . .

But, if we may still trust Boccaccio, "that noble
and most sovereign reason" of Guido was also
"out of tune and harsh" with scrupulous doubt;
"so that lost in speculation, he became abstracted
from men. And since he held somewhat to the
opinion of the Epicureans, gossip among the
vulgar had it that these speculations of his only
went to establish, if established it might be, that
there was no God."

Boccaccio does not call Guido an atheist;
that was mere vulgar gossip. He does not even
declare him a convinced Epicurean, one of those
who with his own father

. . l'anima col corpo morta fanno.

Boccaccio's charge is qualified: "he held somewhat to the opinion of the Epicureans" (*egli alquanto tenea della opinione degli Epicuri*). Dante's commentator, indeed, Benvenuto da Imola, is more categorical and extreme: "Errorem, quem pater habebat ex ignorantia, ipse (Guido) conabatur defendere per scientiam." Benvenuto is even remoter in time, however, than Boccaccio; and his phrasing suggests at least a mere perpetuation of that vulgar gossip which Boccaccio contemptuously records. But can we trust Boccaccio's own testimony?

At least there is no antecedent improbability. Skepticism was common, especially in the highly educated class to which Guido belonged; and it was not unnatural at any rate for him to weigh carefully an opinion held by his own father. Again, there is nothing in either his life or writings to indicate an active faith. Much indeed has been made of his "pilgrimage" to the shrine of St. James at Compostella; but the mood of this was so little serious that a pretty face at Toulouse was enough to change his intention. The ironical sonnet of Muscia of Siena is a hint that his contemporaries could not take him very seriously as a pious pilgrim; and Muscia stressed Guido's excuse for breaking his supposed vow that there was no vow in the case — "*non v'era botio.*" Guido *may* have started in a moment of reaction

from his doubt — does not doubt itself imply a
wavering will? He *may* have left Florence as a
matter of prudence — Corso tried to have him
assassinated on the way as it was. As for his
writings, these, considering the intimate theological
association of the school of Guinizelli, are notice-
ably barren of religious feeling or phrase; and
he certainly scandalized the worthy, if narrow,
Orlandi by his jesting sonnet about the thauma-
turgic shrine of "*my* Lady." The hypothetical
confirmation of Guido's skepticism, on the other
hand, in his "disdain for Virgil," mentioned by
Dante in his answer to the elder Cavalcanti's
question [1] why Dante's "first friend" had not
accompanied him, has been discredited after
twenty years of support by its own proposer,
D'Ovidio. The passage is, to be sure, still a
moot question; and D'Ovidio, even in the zeal
of his recantation, still admits the allegorical
taking of it to be plausible as a secondary intention on Dante's part. In any case, even waiving
the confirmation, the tradition of Guido's skepticism is not impugned; and in view of the per-
sistent tradition, and of the antecedent probability
in its favor, the burden of disproof would seem
to rest on those who reject the tradition. Meanwhile, I propose to test the credibility of the

[1] *Inferno*, x, 60.

tradition by assuming it. If the assumption
proves to be a factor in a coherent and credible
interpretation of Guido's poetry, the credibility
of the assumption proportionately increases.
The argument is, of course, a circle, but I think
not a vicious circle.

There is also another tradition, which happens
likewise to be subsidiary to the same end. As the
one tradition charges Guido with unfaith in religion, so the other charged him with faithlessness
in love. Mr. Maurice Hewlett, in his *Masque of
Dead Florentines*, has seized upon this supposed
fickleness of Guido as Guido's characteristic
trait. Guido is made to say : —

> My way was best.
> From lip to lip I past, from grove to grove :
> I am like Florence ; they call me Light o' Love.

I am dubious indeed about that literal criticism which surmises a "family skeleton" in
every locked sonnet. Heine assuredly reckoned
without his *Scholar* when he complained : —

> Diese Welt glaubt nicht an Flammen,
> Und sie nimmt's für Poesie.

When Guido writes a sonnet describing how Love
had wounded him with three arrows, — *Beauty,
Desire, Hope of Grace*, — it is hardly fair for
Rossetti to entitle his own translation *He speaks*

of a third love of his. Rossetti the scholar
should have known better. Of course Guido is
simply copying a conceit from the *Romance of
the Rose:* the three arrows are three arrows from
the eyes of one lady, not of three ladies. Again,
it is almost worse when poor Guido essays a pretty
pastourelle, which is by definition a gallant adventure between a passing knight and a shepherdess, to discuss the "peccadillo" in a solemn
footnote! Yet Rossetti, himself a poet, does so.
Nay, Guido's latest learned editor, Signor Rivalta, speaks [1] of his singing "anche i suoi desi-
deri meno puri e più umani come nella ballata : —

    In un boschetto trovai pasturella . . ."

This ballata is the *pastourelle* in question. Still,
waiving such pseudo-revelations of a stethoscopic
criticism, there are, considering the meagerness of
Guido's poetical remains, hints enough besides the
mention of several ladies — Mandetta, Pinella,
and by inference her whom Dante calls Giovanna
— to accept with discretion sober Guido Orlandi's
perhaps malicious insinuation, when he inquires
of Guido Cavalcanti concerning the nature, the
effects, the virtues of Love : —

      Io ne domando voi, Guido, di lui :
      odo che molto usate in la sua corte ;

    [1] *Le Rime di Guido Cavalcanti,* Bologna, 1902, p. 23.
    G

and even the cruder implication in Orlandi's boast of his chaster mind : —

> Io per lung' uso disusai lo primo
> amor carnale : non tangio nel limo.

Reckless feudist, unbeliever, "light o' love," squire of dames, profound thinker, gracious gentleman — a perplexing motley of a man; it is no wonder that his poetry, reflecting himself, more easily with its many-faceted light dazzles rather than illumines the understanding. In addition, one has to contend in his more doctrinal pieces, especially in the famous canzone of love, with a rigorous scholastic terminology dovetailed into a most intricate metrical schema, and with a text at the best corrupt. In spots Guido — as we have him — is as hopeless as Persius; yet we may waive these and still venture upon a general interpretation.

In general, Guido's love poems hinge upon two parallel but opposite moods, — a radiant mood of worshipful admiration of his lady, a tragic mood of despair wrought in him by his love of her. His sight of her is a rapture, as in the most magnificent of his sonnets, beginning "Chi è questa che ven" :

> Chi è questa che ven ch' ogn' om la mira
> e fa tremar di chiaritate l' a' re,
> e mena seco amor sì che parlare
> null' omo pote, ma ciascun sospira ?

O Deo, che sembra quando li occhi gira
    dica 'l Amor, ch' i' no 'l savria contare :
    cotanto d' umiltà donna mi pare,
    ch' ogn' altra ver di lei i' la chiam' ira.

Non si poria contar la sua piagenza,
    ch' a lei s' inchina ogni gentil virtute,
    e la beltate per sua dea la mostra.

Non fu sì alta già la mente nostra
    e non si pose in noi tanta salute,
    che propriamente n' aviam canoscenza.[1]

The sonnet is a superb tribute; but it is also
more. It contains, as I conceive, the pivotal
idea in Guido's philosophy of love, — namely,
in the lines describing his mistress as

[1] Lo ! who is this which cometh in men's eyes
    And maketh tremulously bright the air,
    And with her bringeth love so that none there
    Might speak aloud, albeit each one sighs?

Dear God, what seemeth if she turn her eyes
    Let Love's self say, for I in no wise dare :
    Lady of Meekness such, that by compare
    All others as of Wrath I recognize.

Words might not body forth her excellence,
    For unto her inclineth all sweet merit,
    Beauty in her hath its divinity.

Nor was our understanding of degree,
    Nor had abode in us so blest a spirit,
    As might thereof have meet intelligence.

> Lady of Meekness such, that by compare
> All others as of Wrath I recognize.

> (cotanto d' umiltà donna mi pare,
> ch' ogn' altra ver di lei i' la chiam' ira.)

Ira . . . umiltà: wrath . . . meekness — the antithesis dominates Guido's thought. Wrath is in his vocabulary the concomitant of imperfection, of desire; meekness, the concomitant of perfection, of peace. He, the lover, is therefore in a state of wrath; she, the lovable, in a state of meekness, —

> Quiet she, he passion-rent.

The identification of passionate love with a state of wrath is fundamental in Guido's philosophy. It is the germinal idea of the doctrinal canzone beginning "Donna mi prega." In answer to the query as to the where and whence of the passion —

> Là ove si posa e chi lo fa creare —

he declares that

> In quella parte dove sta memora
> prende suo stato, sì formato come
> diaffan da lume, — d'una scuritate
> la qual da Marte vene e fa dimora.[1]

[1] vv. 15–18. I use here as elsewhere the edition of Ercole Rivalta, Bologna, 1902.

"In that part where memory is love has its being;
and, even as light enters into an object to make it
diaphanous, so there enters into the constitution
of love a dark ray from Mars, which abides."
Now Dante conceives love as an emanation from
the star of the third heaven, Venus, along a bright
ray: "I say then that this spirit (*i.e.* of love)
comes upon the "rays of the star" (*i.e.* of the third
heaven, Venus), because you are to know that the
rays of each heaven are the path whereby their
virtue descends upon things that are here below.
And inasmuch as rays are no other than the shining
which cometh from the source of the light through
the air even to the thing enlightened, and the
light is only in that part where the star is, because
the rest of the heaven is diaphanous (that is transparent), I say not that this 'spirit,' to wit this
thought, cometh from their heaven in its totality
but from their star. Which star, by reason of
nobility in them who move it, is of so great virtue
that it has extreme power upon our souls and upon
other affairs of ours," etc.[1] So Dante. Guido,
on the other hand, while accepting the notion of
love as an emanation, holds the emanation to
be rather from the star of the fifth heaven, Mars,
along a dark ray. The power over the soul of
this star is no less extreme than that of Venus;

[1] *Conv.*, II. vii. (Wicksteed's translation.)

only it is, in a sense, a power of darkness rather than of light. It may strike at life itself —

> Di sua potenza segue spesso morte. (v. 35.)

The passion which its influence excites passes all normal bounds in any case, destroying all healthful equilibrium : —

> L'esser è quando lo voler è tanto
> ch' oltra misura di natura torna :
> poi non s' adorna di riposo mai.
> Move cangiando color riso e pianto
> e la figura con paura storna. . . .[1] (vv. 43–47.)

Finally, — and here we reach the gist of the matter, — the influence of the choleric planet engenders sighs and fiery wrath in the lover, impotent to reach the ever-receding goal of his desire (*non fermato loco*) :—

> La nova qualità move sospiri
> e vol ch' om miri in non fermato loco
> destandos' ira, la qual manda foco.[2]

This strangely pessimistic reading of love seems to have struck at least one of Guido's contem-

---

[1] Its essence is when the passionate will
Beyond the measure of natural pleasure goes :
Then with repose forever is unblest.
Still fickle, smiles in tears it can fulfil,
And on the face leave pallid trace of woes.

[2] To sighs the new-given quality invites ;
Through it man sights an ever-shifting aim,
Till in him wrath is kindled, darting flame.

poraries with indignant surprise, not only at the
apparent slight upon love, but also at the silence
seeming to give assent of other poets, especially
of Dante. Cecco d' Ascoli, in his *Acerba*, iii, 1,
denies that so sweet a thing as love could emanate
from the planet Mars, seeing that from that planet
rather "proceeds violence with wrath" (*procede
l'impeto con l'ire*) ; wherefore : —

> Errando scrisse Guido Cavalcanti. . . .
> qui ben mi sdegna lo tacer di Danti.

In fact, Dante, in the sonnet in the sixteenth
chapter of the *New Life*, apparently alludes
sympathetically to Guido's dark rays of love —

> Spesse fiate vegnommi a la mente
> l'oscure qualità ch' Amor mi dona —

and proceeds to describe, though not by this
name, just such a "state of wrath" in himself
as Guido believes inseparable from love. With
Dante, of course, the mood is but passing. For
him love is in its essence a beneficent power.

For Guido also it might seem that this tragic
wrath of desire is not incurable. There is a power
in meekness to overcome wrath and to subdue
wrath also to meekness. And the meek one is
impelled to exercise this power, to confer this
boon, by pity for the one suffering in wrath. ˙It
is the failure to follow this blessed impulse for

which Guido reproaches his lady in the octave
of the sonnet beginning "Un amoroso sguardo,"
when he says that she is one

> . . . for whom availeth not
> Nor grace nor pity nor the suffering state. . . .
> (. . . verso cui non vale
> Merzede nè pietà nè star soffrente. . . .)

Meekness, grace, pity, the suffering state of
wrath — the terms have a scriptural sound, and
of right; for they are actually scriptural analogies
applied to love. Precisely this poetical analogy
was the innovation of Guido Guinizelli, whom
Dante called "father of me and of my betters,"
— of which last Guido Cavalcanti was in Dante's
mind first, if not alone. Before Guinizelli Italian
poets had accepted the other analogy of the
troubadours of Provence, which applied to love
the canon of feudal homage. For these the lady
of desire was as the haughty baron to whom they
owed servile fealty, and whose inaccessible mood
was not of gentle meekness but of cruel pride,
claiming willfully of her vassal perhaps life itself.
But feudalism and its harsh canon of service were
alien to the Italian communes; Italian poetry
built upon an analogy with it must needs be an
affectation. These burgher poets were only play
knights; these frank Tuscan and Lombard girls
were only play barons. Affectation, the pen

following not the dictation of the feelings but of
hearsay feelings, — this is the precise charge
which Dante, from the standpoint of the "sweet
new style," brings against the older style.[1] But
if as free burghers Italians could not really feel
the alien mood of feudal homage, yet as Christian
gentlemen they could, and should, sanctify their
love of women with the mood of religious awe.
There need be no affectation in that. Free
burghers, they recognized no temporal overlord,
no absolute baron; Catholics, they did believe
in, and might with sincerity worship, ministering
angels — "donne angelicate," the *meek* ones
whom, as the Psalmist had declared, the Lord
has beautified with salvation.

Guido therefore can no more worthily praise
his mistress than by calling her his "Lady of
Meekness." Indeed, by further analogy he sets
her above the angels themselves; for the Christ
himself had said: "*Mitis sum et humilis corde* —
I am meek and lowly in heart." For himself,
"passion-rent" in his love, the poet speaks as
St. Paul, — "we . . . had our conversation . . .
in the lusts of our flesh, fulfilling the desires of
the flesh and of the mind; and were by nature the
children of wrath (*filii iræ*)." And the *merzede*,
the "grace," for which he sues — solution of

[1] *Purgatorio*, xxiv, 49 seq.

wrath by the spirit of meekness — is again in
accord with Paul's promise to these very "children
of wrath," — "By grace are ye saved through
faith," — faith, that is, in loving and serving the
one divinity as the other.

This is pious doctrine indeed for the fighting
cavalier, skeptic, Lovelace, I have in a measure
assumed Guido to be. Is then his love creed also
a pose, worse than the apes of Provence whom
Dante exposed, because he thus adds hypocrisy
to affectation? Well, if so, the same Dante
would hardly have hailed him as "first friend"
in life and master after Guinizelli in poetry, nor
have outraged the memory of Beatrice by associat-
ing her in the *New Life* with Guido's lady Joan.

The solution of the apparent antinomy lies in
the meaning for Guido of that *merzede*, that
"grace," the granting of which by the lady, the
meek one, might appease the lover, the one in
"wrath." The term itself — Italian *merzede* or
English "grace" — has a fourfold significance
according as it is a function of the lady, of the
lover, or of the reciprocal relationship between
them. "Grace" in her signifies her beatitude,
her "meekness;" in him, his "merit" which
through faith and loving service deserves the
boon, or "grace," of her condescension to redeem
him from his "state of wrath," for which con-

descension it would be befitting him to render thanks, "yield graces," — a phrase now obsolete in English but used by Dante, — *render mercede.* Of this fourfold intention of the term the one fundamentally doubtful is the "grace" which is constituted by the act of condescension of the lady: what then is the grace or boon that the lover asks and hopes? In other words, what is the end of desire?

The answer is no mystery. The end of desire is always possession, in one sense or another, of the thing desired. In the practical sense possession of the loved one means union, physical or social, or both, sacramentally recognized, in marriage; but the sacrament of marriage allows a more mystical sense, presenting the ideal, hardly realizable on earth, of a spiritual union which is also a unity of two in one: —

> The single pure and perfect animal,
> The two-cell'd heart beating with one full stroke,
> Life.

So Tennyson modernly; but more in accord with the metaphysical mood of Guido is the old Elizabethan phrasing: —

> So they loved, as love in twain
> Had the essence but in one;
> Two distincts, division none:
> Number there in love was slain.

To the "gentle heart" there is no love but highest love; there is no union but perfect union, wherein two shall

> Be one, and one another's all.

Until the "gentle heart" may attain to that perfect union its desire is unappeased, its "wrath" unsubdued. Tennyson premises it for the right marriage; but there is ever the doubter ready to remark that if such marriages are really made in heaven, they certainly are kept there. Human sympathy cannot quite bridge the span between two souls: self remains self; and though hands meet and lips touch and wills accord, there is always something deeper still, inexpressible, unreachable.

> Yes! in the sea of life enisled,
> With echoing straits between us thrown,
> Dotting the shoreless watery wild,
> We mortal millions live *alone*.

In vain, says Aristophanes in Plato's *Banquet*, in vain, "after the division (of the primeval man-woman in one), the two parts of man, each desiring his other half, came together, and threw their arms about one another eager to grow into one. . . ." True, Aristophanes in effect goes on, Zeus in pity consoled the loneliness of dissevered "man-woman" by physical union; but that consolation the "gentle heart" must forever regard as of itself inadequate and unworthy.

There is indeed a solution. Guinizelli and Dante read further into the *Banquet* of Plato — or into the Christian doctrine built upon that — to where the wise woman of Mantineia reveals the mysteries of a love extending into a mystic otherworld — at least so Christians read her teaching — where in the bosom of God all become as one. There "wrath" is resolved into "meekness" perfectly.

The love of Guinizelli, and of Dante, was the love of happier men of which Arnold speaks : —

> Of happier men — for they, at least,
> Have *dream'd* two human hearts might blend
> In one, and were through faith released
> From isolation without end
> Prolong'd.

But if Guido, even as Arnold, lacked this faith, doubted this mystic otherworld whither therefore he might not accompany his first friend to find his Giovanna, as Dante his Beatrice, perfect in meekness, purged of all wrath, and to learn from her release hereafter from the dividing flesh, union at last with her spirit at peace? — if he was of those, even uncertainly wavered with those, who

> . . . l' anima col corpo morta fanno? —

then indeed for him, in degree as his desire was

ideally exalted, so its grace, its *merzede*, became
an irony, a tragic paradox. His must be a passionate loneliness forever teased by an illusion,
a phantom mate of its own conjuring. And I
at least so understand the concluding words of
the canzone : —

> For di colore d'esser è diviso,
>> assiso in mezzo scuro luce rade :
>> for d'onne fraude dice, degno in fede,
>> che solo di costui nasce mercede.[1]

That is, the only love of which grace is born, entire
possession granted, is love of the dim immaterial
idea, — "*la figlia della sua mente, l'amorosa idea*,"
as Leopardi calls it. Ixion embraces his Cloud.
Guido's lady's desirable perfection, her "meekness," exists not in her, but in his glorified ideal
of her, "dispossessed" as that is "of color of being."
Therefore Guido's mood is essentially one with
Leopardi's when the latter exclaims : —

> Solo il mio cor piaceami, e col mio core
> In un perenne ragionar sepolto,
> Alla guardia seder del mio dolore.[2]

---

[1] Of color of being Love is dispossessed.
At rest in shadow space it cancels light.
Without false sleight saith a faithworthy one,
That from it only is the guerdon won.

[2] Only my heart pleased me, and, with my heart
In a communing without cease absorbed,
Still to keep watch and ward o'er my own smart.

Guido has himself described with quaint "pre-raphaelite" symbolism the process of progressive detachment of the ideal from the real in the ballata beginning "Veggio ne gli occhi."

> Cosa m' avien quand' i' le son presente
>   ch' i' no la posso a lo 'ntelletto dire:
>   veder mi par de la sua labbia uscire
>   una sì bella donna, che la mente
>   comprender no la può; che 'nmantenente
>   ne nasce un' altra di bellezza nova,
>   da la qual par ch' una stella si mova
>   e dica: la salute tua è apparita.[1]

The imagery here is manifestly in accord with contemporary pictorial symbolism, in which souls as living manikins issue forth from the lips of the dead; but the significance of the passage is, I take it, at one with that of the so-called Platonic "ladder of love" by which through successive abstractions the pure idea, the intelligible virtue, is reached. The following stanza in the same ballata again defines this "virtue" as "meekness," and again declares it to be merely "intelligible,"

---

[1] Something befalleth me when she is by
    Which unto reason can I not make clear:
    Meseems I see forth through her lips appear
    Lady of fairness such that faculty
    Man hath not to conceive; and presently
    Of this one springs another of new grace,
    Who to a star then seemeth to give place,
    Which saith: Thy blessedness hath been with thee.

> for di colore d' esser . . . diviso,
>   assiso in mezzo scuro luce rade;

only instead of the metaphysical directness of
the canzone, the poet employs the theological
tropes of the *dolce stil.*

> Là dove questa bella donna appare
>   s' ode una voce che le ven davanti,
>   e par che d' umiltà 'l su' nome canti
>   sì dolcemente, che s' i' 'l vo' contare
>   sento che 'l su' valor mi fa tremare.
>   E movonsi ne l' anima sospiri
>   che dicon : guarda, se tu costei miri
>   vedrai la sua vertù nel ciel salita.[1]

And now the tragic note in Guido's is explained.
It is neither the polite fiction, the "pathetic
fallacy" of the Sicilian school, nor yet the quickly
passing shadow of this life set between Dante and
the sun of his desire.

> La tua magnificenza in me custodi,
>   Sì che l' anima mia che fatta hai sana,
>   Piacente a te dal corpo si disnodi.
> Cosi orai . . .[2]

[1] There where this gentle lady comes in sight
    Is heard a voice which moveth her before
    And, singing, seemeth that Meekness to adore
    Which is her name, so sweetly, that aright
    I may not tell for trembling at its might.
    And then within my soul there gather sighs
    Which say : Lo ! unto this one turn thine eyes :
    To heaven her virtue wingeth visibly.

[2] *Paradiso,* xxxi, 88–91.

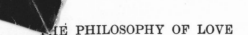

"So I prayed," writes Dante, triumphant in expectation; but for those

Che l 'anima col corpo morta fanno,

there could be health of soul neither now nor hereafter. Wherefore Guido's text in the analysis of his own passion is in all literalness the words of the Preacher, — "All his days . . . he eateth in *darkness,* and he hath much *sorrow* and *wrath* in his sickness." Until Guido prays indeed for release in death, not triumphantly as Dante, but piteously, in the spirit of Leopardi's words in *Amore Morte:* —

Nova, sola, infinita
Felicità . . . il suo (the lover's) pensier figura:
Ma per cagion di lei grave procella
Presentendo in suo cor, brama quiete,
Brama raccorsi in porto
Dinanzi al fier disio,
Che già, rugghiando, intorno intorno oscura.[1]

Poi, quando tutto avvolge
La formidabil possa,
E fulmina nel cor l'invitta cura,

[1] Not only are Guido and Leopardi saying the same thing in effect, but even their figures of speech are in accord. There is evident similarity of symbolism between the soul-darkening storm blast of the one and the soul-darkening Martian ray of the other; although possibly the medieval poet may have conceived his "dark ray" as a real phenomenon.

H

> Quante volte implorata
> Con desiderio intenso,
> Morte, sei tu dall' affanoso amante![1]

Precisely in this mood Guido invokes death : —

> Morte gientil, rimedio de' cattivi,
>   merzè merzè a man giunte ti cheggio :
>   vienmi a vedere e prendimi, chè peggio
>   mi face amor : chè mie' spiriti vivi
> son consumati e spenti sì, che quivi,
>   dov' i' stava gioioso, ora mi veggio
>   in parte, lasso, là dov' io posseggio
>   pena e dolor con pianto : e vuol ch' arrivi
> ancòra in più di mal s' esser più puote ;
>   perchè tu, morte, ora valer mi puoi
>   di trarmi de le man di tal nemico.
> Aime ! lasso quante volte dico :
>   amor, perchè fai mal pur sol a' tuoi
>   come quel de lo 'nferno che i percuote?[2]

[1] New, infinite, unique
Felicity . . . he pictures to his mind :
And yet because of it the wrath of storm
Foreboding in his heart, he longs for calm,
Longs for the quiet haven
Far from that fierce desire,
Which even now, rumbling, darkens all around.

      Then, when o'erwhelmeth him
The fury of its might,
And in his heart thunders unconquerable care,
How many times he calls
In agony of need,
Death, upon thee in his extremity !

[2] Gentle death, refuge of th' unfortunate,
    Mercy, mercy with clasp'd hands I implore :

At other times Guido describes the combat to the death between his "spirits" of life and love. He enlarges his canvas and, calling to aid a whole *dramatis personœ* of the various "souls" and "animal spirits" of scholastic psychology, objectifies his mood into miniature epic and drama. This mythology of the inner world arose naturally enough to mind from the ambiguity of the term "spirits," meaning at once bodily humors and bodiless but personal creatures; and in Guido's delicate handling the symbolism is singularly effective. Only by exaggeration of imitation did it grow stale and ludicrous, meriting the jibes of Onesto da Bologna at such *"sporte piene di spiriti."* The following curiously rhymed sonnet may illustrate his manner in this kind : —

> Look down upon me, take me, since more sore
> Hath been love's dealing: in so evil state
>
> Are brought the spirits of my life, that late
> Where I stood joyous, now I stand no more,
> But find me where, alas ! I have much store
> Of pain and grief with weeping: and my fate
>
> Yet wills more woe if more of woe might be;
> Wherefore canst thou, death, now avail alone
> To loose the clutch of such an enemy.
>
> How many times I say, Ah woe is me !
> Love, wherefore only wrongest thou thine own,
> As He of Hell from his wrings misery ?

> L' anima mia vilment' è sbigotita
>   de la battaglia ch' ell' ave dal core,
>   che, s' ella sente pur un poco amore
>   più presso a lui che nou sole, la more.
>
> Sta come quella che non à valore,
>   ch' è per temenza da lo cor partita:
>   e chi vedesse com' ell' è fuggita
>   diria per certo: questi non à vita.
>
> Per gli occhi venne la battaglia in pria,
>   che ruppe ogni valore immantenente
>   sì, che del colpo fu strutta la mente.
>
> Qualunqu' è quei che più allegrezza sente,
>   se dedesse li spirti fuggir via,
>   di grande sua pietate piangeria.[1]

It transpires then for Guido as for Leopardi
that the only grace, the only boon of peace, to
which love leads is death; and so is verified the

[1] The spirit of my life is sore bested
        By battle whereof at heart she heareth cry,
        So, that if but a little closer by
        Love than his wont she feeleth, she must die.

She is as one dejected utterly;
        The heart she hath deserted in her dread:
        And who perceiveth how that she is fled,
        Saith of a certainty: This man is dead.

First through the eyes swept down the battle-tide,
        Which broke incontinently all defense,
        And by its wrath wrecked the intelligence.

Whoever he that most of joy hath sense,
        Yet if he saw the spirits scattered wide,
        In his excess of pity must have sighed.

warning of those who came to meet him when he
first entered the court of love : —

> Quando mi vider, tutti con pietanza
>   dissermi : fatto se' di tal servente
>   che mai non dei sperare altro che morte.[1]

In reality, he knows the futility of any appeal
to his lady for aid. She is indeed the innocent
occasion of his suffering, but of it she is a mere
passive spectator, hardly understanding it, and
certainly helpless to relieve it; and so Guido
himself describes her in the sonnet beginning
"S' io prego questa donna."   In the midst of
his agony,

> Allora par che ne la mente piova
>   una figura di donna pensosa,
>   che vegna per veder morir lo core.[2]

Here then at last we find the explanation of
his interpretation of Dante's sonnet, when he
said that love fed Dante's heart to his lady,

> vegendo
> che vostra donna la morte chedea.

She claimed its death not willfully indeed, as the
capricious mistress of Ulrich von Lichtenstein

----

[1] When they beheld me, unto me all cried
    Pitiful : bondman art thou made of one
    Such that for nought else mayst thou look but death.

[2] "Into my mind then seems it that there rays a figure of
a pensive lady, coming to behold my heart die."

"claimed" his mutilation, but innocently, un-
wittingly, in that her beauty was as a firebrand,
her perfection, her "meekness," a goal of unavail-
ing consuming desire. She is helpless to relieve
him, because — and here is the core of the matter
— it is not she, not the real woman, that he loves,
but that idealization of her which exists only in
his own mind —

> for di colore d'esser è diviso,
> assiso in mezzo scuro luce rade.

Compared with this glorified phantom "nel ciel
(that is, into the intelligible world) salita," the real
woman also is but "ira," wrath and imperfection.
So he pines for his lady of dreams, who thus a
ghostly "vampire" feeds upon his human heart;
but the real woman, "the woman who does not
understand," is no longer of moment to him.
She is, as it were, but the nameless model to his
artist mind. When that has drawn from her all
that is of fitness for its masterpiece, it straight-
way leaves her for another otherwise completing
the ideal type. Giovanni passes; Mandetta
arrives.

> Una giovane donna di Tolosa
> bell' e gentil, d'onesta leggiadria,
> tant' è diritta e simigliante cosa,
> ne' suoi dolci occhi, de la donna mia,

ch' è fatta dentro al cor desiderosa
    l' anima in guisa, che da lui si svia
    e vanne a lei ; ma tant' è paurosa,
    che no le dice di qual donna sia.

Quella la mira nel su' dolce sguardo,
    ne lo qual face rallegrare amore,
    perchè v' è dentro la sua donna dritta.

Po' torna, piena di sospir, nel core,
    ferita a morte d' un tagliente dardo,
    che questa donna nel partir li gitta.[1]

Plainly it is not of Giovanni, nor of any actual
woman, but of his ideal woman, of whom Giovanni
herself was but a reminiscence, that Mandetta

---

[1] A lady of Toulouse, young and most fair,
    Gentle, and of unwanton joyousness,
    So is the very image and impress,
    In her sweet eyes, of one I name in prayer,

That my soul's wish is more than it can bear:
    Wherefore it 'scapeth from the heart's duress
    And cometh unto her ; yet for distress
    What lady it obeys may not declare.

She looketh on it with her gentle mien,
    Whereunto by the will of love it yearns,
    Because that lady there it may perceive.

Then to the heart it, full of sighs, returns,
    Unto death wounded by an arrow keen,
    The which this lady loosed when taking leave.

reminds him. In her turn Mandetta will pass also. Then will come Pinella, or another — what does it matter? What cared Zeuxis for any one of his five Crotonian maidens, once each in her turn had supplied that particular trait of loveliness which only she, perhaps, had to offer, but had to offer only?

> Mentre ch' alla beltà, ch' i' viddi in prima
>   Apresso l' alma, che per gli ochi vede,
>   L' inmagin dentro crescie, e quella cede
>   Quasi vilmente e senza alcuna stima.[1]

The words are Michelangelo's, but the idea is in effect Guido's. And it is an idea which, I think, renders perfectly compatible in him constancy in ideal love with inconstancy in real loves. To keep faith with perfection is to break faith with imperfection. The love of Guido brooked no compromise. The perfect one might be unattainable in this life; perfect union with her, even if found, might be impossible in this life; there might be no other life than this so marred by the perpetual "state of wrath" to which his impossible desire in its impotence doomed him; yet

---

[1] While to the beauty which I first regarded
    I turn my soul, that through mine eyes perceiveth,
    Within my soul that beauty's image liveth,
    Itself as base and worthless is discarded.

nevertheless Guido was willing to be damned for the greater glory of Love.

In conclusion, I would quote a passage from the elegy to *Aspasia* of Leopardi, which puts into modern phrasing exactly what I conceive to be Guido's intention, obscured as that is for us by its scholastic terminology and its mixture of chivalric and obsolete psychological imagery. Especially I would call attention to the precisely similar way in which Leopardi, like Guido, combines in his mood the loftiest idealization of Woman with the most contemptuous conception of women. So Hamlet insults, even while he adores. Dante too had his cynical time, to judge from Beatrice's immortal rebuke, — when he

> . . . volse i passi suoi per via non vera,
> Imagini di ben seguendo false.

But Dante was saved from ultimate cynicism, ultimate unfaith, by the promise of perfect union with his ideal in paradise. That promise Guido, like Leopardi, rejected.

Here is Leopardi's confession : —

> Raggio divino al mio pensiero apparve,
> Donna, la tua beltà.   Simile effeto
> Fan la bellezza e i musicali accordi,
> Ch' alto mistero d' ignorati Elisi
> Paion sovente rivelar.   Vagheggia

Il piagato mortal quindi la figlia
Della sua mente, l' amorosa idea,
Che gran parte d' Olimpo in sè racchiude,
Tutta al volto, ai costumi, alla favella
Pari alla donna che il rapito amante
Vagheggiare ed amar confuso estima.
Or questa egli non già, ma quella, ancora
Nei corporali amplessi, inchina ed ama.
Alfin l'errore e gli scambiati oggetti
Conoscendo, s' adira . . .

("*S' adira!*" — "is wrathful" — Leopardi's very words form a gloss to Guido's. But as little as Guido's is Leopardi's wrath directed against the real woman, innocent occasion of his illusion and disillusion. Leopardi continues : —)

    . . . e spesso incolpa
La donna a torto. A quella eccelsa imago
Sorge di rado il femminile ingegno ;
E ciò che inspira ai generosi amanti
La sua stessa beltà, donna non pensa.
Nè comprender potria. . . .

("The woman who does not understand"!)

    . . . Non cape in quelle
Anguste fronti ugual concetto. E male
Al vivo sfolgorar di quegli sguardi
Spera l' uomo ingannato, e mal richiede
Sensi profondi, sconosciuti, e molto
Più che virili, in chi dell' uomo al tutto
Da nature è minor. Che se più molli

E più tenui le membra, essa la mente
Men capace e men forte anco riceve.[1]

So the idealist skeptic of the nineteenth century
aligns himself with the idealist skeptic of the
thirteenth, even to that last truly medieval
touch — *confusio hominis est femina.* And, if

[1] A ray celestial to my thought appeared,
Lady, thy loveliness.   Similar effects
Have beauty and those harmonies of music
Which the high mystery of Edens unexplored
Seem ofttimes to illumine.   Even so
Enamored man upon the daughter broods
Of his own fancy, the amorous idea,
Which great part of Olympus comprehends,
In feature all, in manner, and in speech
Unto the woman like, whom, rapturous man,
In his false lights he seems to see and love.
Yet her he doth not, but that other, even
In corporal embracings, crave and love.
Until, his error and the intent transferred
Perceiving, he grows wrathful; and oft blames
With wrong the woman.   To that ideal height
Rarely indeed the wit of woman rises;
And that which is in gentle hearts inspired
By her own beauty, woman dreams not of,
Nor yet might understand.   No room have those
Too straitened foreheads for such thoughts.   And fondly
Upon the spirited flashing of that glance
Builds the infatuate man, and fondly seeks
Meanings profound, undreamt of, and much more
Than masculine, in one than man in all
By kind inferior.   For if more tender,
More delicate of limb, so with a mind
Less broad, less vigorous is she endowed.

I have not somewhere gone off on a tangent, I have described my circle. Guido's philosophy of love at least fits with the hypothesis of his skepticism, and a practical consequence of both would be that actual fickleness of heart to which tradition again bears witness.

GUIDO CAVALCANTI'S ODE OF LOVE

THE following translation is an attempt to render as literally as possible in the original meter the famous philosophical poem of Dante's "first friend." The rendering itself, with the notes, implies necessarily an interpretation of Guido's philosophy.

The Ode itself probaby is in answer to the following sonnet, addressed, as the custom was, to Cavalcanti by a fellow-poet, Guido Orlandi.

GUIDO ORLANDI TO GUIDO CAVALCANTI

Tell me, where is Love born and of what sire?
Is't substance, quality, or remembrance, pray?
What is its natural place, where it holds sway?
Fancy of eye is it, or heart's desire?
From what derives its temper or its ire?
How is it felt as flame that wastes away?
Also I ask, upon what does it prey?
How, when, and over whom has it empire?
What sort of thing, I say, is Love? has't feature?

109

Wears it its own shape, or some counterfeit?
And is it life, this Love, or is it death?
Who serves it, should know somewhat of its nature:
Wherefore I ask you, Guido, touching it:
You're in its service seasoned, rumor saith.

ODE OF LOVE

By Cavalcanti

I

A Lady entreats me; wherefore I will tell
Of a quality too frequently malign,
Yet so divine that men have called it Love:
Thus may the truth whatever doubt dispel.
Adept I ask unto this task of mine,   5
For my design, I fear me, is above
His wit that is at heart of base degree.
For me proof philosophic is defined,
Else disinclined I feel me to recite
Where Love has place; created by what might;

1. *Lady.* In *Convito*, iii, 14, Dante interprets the *donna
gentil* of his *canzone* as "a soul noble in intellect and free in
the exercise of its own proper power, which is reason." Possibly, therefore, we may understand by the "Lady" who
entreats Cavalcanti, the rational soul, or intelligence, of
Orlandi.

2. *Quality.* An *accidente* is a contingent quality. Cavalcanti uses the term *qualità* for love in l. 50.

And what its virtue is; and potency;   11
Verity essential; motions of what kind;
Its name assigned as Love for what delight;
And if it may be manifest to sight.

II

In that part where the memory resides   15
It makes appearance; as transparence shows
Through which light flows, so Love its form ac-
     quires,
From shadow cast by Mars, the which abides.
Created hence; nature of sense bestows

15. *Where the memory resides.* *I.e.* the sensitive soul,
according to Aristotle, where the image of the loved one is
preserved; hence, modernly speaking, the imagination.

16–18. The lovable image is conceived as, so to speak,
a silhouette in black upon the screen of the imagination, so
symbolizing the "malignity" of love (cf. l. 2). This "malignity" is further explained by deriving the "shadow" from
Mars, the planet of wrath and perturbation. Cecco d' Ascoli
in his *Acerba*, iii, 1, takes issue with this derivation of love,
and reproves Dante for failing also to object. In fact, Dante
in *Convito*, iii, 19, does recant his own previous account of
love of "malign" (*fero*): that view "sprang," he says, "from
the infirmity of my mind which was impassioned by excessive
longing." In *Convito*, ii, 7, he derives love from the bright
radiance of Venus. Cavalcanti, however, makes the very
essence of love "excessive longing" (cf. ll. 43, 44).

19. *Created hence.* Since love is excited by an outside
force, *i.e.* literally or symbolically the influence of the planet
Mars, it is not an original and permanent quality of the soul,
but contingent (*accidente*) upon the action of that force.

Its name, and pose of soul, and heart's desire. 20
It comes from visible form, which, apprehended,
Ascended into passive intellect,
There, as affect, maintains its tenancy.
Never it works in that part injury.
And since from finite kind 'tis not descended,
Unended is its radiant effect. 26
Nor wears aspect of joy but reverie,
For may not enter there affinity.

19, 20. *Nature of sense*, etc. Love originates in the sensitive soul, and so has the same name and character and desire
as sensual passion, though its object is quite different. The
aim of all love is union with the thing beloved; but whereas
sensual passion desires only physical union, love in the proper
sense desires spiritual union. So Dante (*Convito*, iii, 2):
"Love, truly taken and subtly considered, is nought else than a
spiritual union of the soul and of the loved thing."

21–23. The "visible form" or idea incarnate, is "apprehended," that is, its pure form or idea is abstracted from the
material thing, and taken up into the passive intellect, or
intellective memory, where it remains as a dominating ideal.

24. The action of this amorous ideal is not directly mental,
i.e. ratiocinative or discursive, but obsessive of the attention
and will: to speak modernly, it becomes a "fixed idea."

25, 26. Being of a pure form, or idea, which as infinite
cannot be completely possessed by a finite being, love is never
inactive through satiety.

27, 28. Love cannot enjoy its ideal in the sense of fruition,
as just said; its mood is an entranced contemplation of that
ideal, a ravishment away from self toward it. Cavalcanti
intends the same as the platonic "ecstasy." The "affinity"
is the "ideal" as it exists objectively in the intelligible world,
according to Plato, or in the "active intelligence" according
to Aristotle. (Cf. l. 75 and comment.)

III

It is not virtue, but from that proceeds
Which is perfection, in complexion withal   30
Not rational, but feeling, I attest.
The judgment Love against well-being leads,
For ravishments intelligence enthrall.
Discernment small it has where vice is guest.
Often there follows from its puissance death,   35
If wrath o'ermuch the faculty dismay
Which of the way adversative is ward:
Not that with nature Love hath disaccord;
But when to perfect good lies not its path,
Who saith that life is his is led astray,   40
Lacking the stay which makes him his own lord.
Nor less avails Love though it be ignored.

29–31. Virtue, moral or intellectual, is a rational perfection;
love is not rational, but "feels." Its object, however, is not
a sensation, but an idea; and to "feel" an idea is, modernly
speaking, to "intuit." Love, then, is an intuitive perfection.

32, 33. Its intuitions of its ideal act, as said before, like
"fixed ideas," dominating the judgment against the welfare
of the organism; the mind is in a state of ecstatic brooding
(*intenzione*).

35–37. Wrath (*ira*) (cf. ll. 51, 52), occasioned by the im-
possibility of fruition (cf. l. 28), may fatally impair the vital
faculties. Cf. the exclamation of Dante's "natural spirit"
at the first appearance of Beatrice, *Heu miser! quia frequenter
impeditus ero deinceps.*

38–41. It is not love that works against nature, for, on
the contrary, love is the very principle which moves nature;
but it is, as said, the inability of love to reach its "perfect

I

IV

Its essence is whenas the passionate will
Beyond the measure of natural pleasure goes;
Then with repose forever is unblest.   45
Still fickle, smiles in tears it can fulfill,
And on the face leave pallid trace of woes.
Brief are its throes.   Yet chiefly manifest
Thou shalt observe it in the nobly wise.
To sighs the new-given quality invites;   50
Through it man sights an ever-shifting aim,
Till in him wrath is kindled, darting flame.
Conceive it none save one its puissance tries.
Complies it never though it still incites;
And no delights one seeketh in its name,   55
Neither great wisdom, sooth — or small — to
        frame.

V

A glance Love draws from like-attempered heart
Which seeming right to all delight implies.
In secret guise Love comes not, so declared.

good," which causes the "wrath" which deprives the lover of
the self-control without which self-preservation is impossible.

43, 44. Natural pleasure, or instinct, is of the attainable;
the essence of love, for Cavalcanti, is that it seeks the unattainable.   (Cf. comment on ll. 16–18.)

48, 49. Obviously only the few are capable of such love.

51. *An ever-shifting aim*.   *I.e.* again the unattainable
idea, or ideal.

57–59. Requited love is revealed through the meeting of
eyes, and seems to promise satisfaction.

Indeed not scornful beauty is the dart.   60
For that way led desire through dread is wise,
But merit lies with spirit that is snared.
And not to sight is Love made manifest,
For by its test o'ertaken man falls white;
And, hears one right that form is seen by none, 65
Then least by him that is by Love undone.
Of color of being Love is dispossessed.
At rest in shadow space it cancels light.
Without false sleight saith a faith-worthy one,
That from it only is the guerdon won.   70

VI

Ode, thou mayst go thy ways, unfaltering,
Where pleases thee : I have thee so adorned
That never scorned shall be thy reasoning
By such as bring to thee intelligence :
To bide with others maks't thou no pretence.   75

60–62. Scornful beauty repels love, at least when grown
wary through experience. Genuine love invites requital.
Cf. Dante : *Amor che a nullo amato amar perdona.*

63–68. But true love is of the invisible idea, which, were it
to appear in its reality to mortal man, would overwhelm him
utterly ; of it the lover's ideal is but the reflection.

67, 68. Again, insistence on the supersensuousness of
love's object, which reflected darkly in the soul, darkens all.

70. This supersensuous ideal is the guerdon the lover seeks,
and can win only through loss of his separateness from its
abode in the active intelligence, that is, by loss of his separable
self-consciousness. "He that loseth his life shall find it."

BENIVIENI'S ODE OF LOVE AND SPENSER'S "FOWRE HYMNES"

JERØME BENIVIENI's *Canzona dello Amore celeste et divino* was published about 1488. Benivieni was a disciple of Marsilio Ficino, and his Ode was based on Ficino's neo-platonic commentary on Plato's *Symposium*. To the Ode itself, Benivieni's friend, Pico della Mirandola, contributed an elaborate commentary, treating the poem as a *summa* of platonism, as reconstructed by the Florentine cenacle. So advertised, the Ode with its critical apparatus went through a number of editions, and became internationally celebrated. Pico himself regarded it as a complement to Cavalcanti's famous ode beginning *Donna mi prega;* and failing to perceive any doctrinal difference, held Cavalcanti's ode to have dealt with profane, Benivieni's with sacred, love. In fact, however, each poet treated love of both kinds, but Cavalcanti in the light of Aristotle interpreted by Averroës, Benivieni in the light of Plato interpreted by Ficino after Plotinus.

116

The influence of Florentine neo-platonism upon Spenser, and especially upon his *Fowre Hymnes*, has been generally recognized, and recently summarized.[1] "The most probable channels of this influence," says Miss Winstanley, "were Marsilio Ficino and Giordano Bruno." In the light of the evidences presented in the following notes, however, it would appear that the direct "channel" was Benivieni, although, no doubt, Spenser knew Ficino and Bruno as well. The term "Hymne" is used by Spenser in the sense of the Greek ὕμνος, — song or pæan in honor of a god or hero, especially as colored philosophically in the so-called "Orphic Hymns," or τελεταί, hymns of initiation into the mysteries of the Hellenic religion. In this sense, the "Fowre Hymnes" exactly correspond to the philosophic canzoni of Cavalcanti and Benivieni. The term itself Spenser may have taken directly from the Greek, or have borrowed from Ronsard, by whom it had been shortly before revived.

The two original *Hymnes in Honour of Love* and of *Beautie*, taken together, suggest briefly the dialectic ascent from sensual to intellectual love as it is developed in Benivieni's Canzone, only Spenser's plan of two separate pæans causes

[1] *The Fowre Hymnes*, ed. by Lilian Winstanley, Cambridge (Eng.), 1907.

some repetition and rearrangement. Broadly speaking, the first Hymne carries the dialectic course only as far as the fifth grade of love,[1] that is, to Intellectual Beauty as realizable by the mind in its individual and temporal nature; the second Hymne, however, rises in brief suggestion to the sixth and — short of the mystical "ecstasy" — last grade. Both Spenser and Benivieni barely hint at the seventh grade, in which the soul is merged with God. Spenser is less austerely systematic than Benivieni, introducing — at times from Pico's commentary — much didactic and illustrative matter; and he hints in the beginning and end of each Hymne at his own very present experience as a scorned lover. Spenser as usual is not content to ride one Pegasus at a time; and so often spurs

Forse di là dal destinato corso

of his model; yet we can, if I mistake not, "without an hound" Benivieni's fine Italian footing trace.

The two later Hymnes purge away all suggestion of romantic love, and develop at length the four higher grades of the soul's reascent to God. Thus the *Fowre Hymnes* really constitute one complete doctrinal poem. Benivieni's neo-platon-

[1] See notes to Benivieni's Ode, stanzas vii–viii.

ism is harmonized with calvinism. The third
Hymne presents the *man*-Christ as the exemplar
of the moral service of true love; the fourth
Hymne promises the *God*-Christ as the mystic
reward of the true lover. "Sapience," the promised "bride" of the soul, represents the God-
Christ in the distinct, yet mystically identical,
person of the Holy Ghost, conceived as feminine
as the gnostics had conceived the *Pneuma*, or
Holy Spirit, and given the place and function of
the *Venus Urania* of the neo-platonists. "Sapience" is given the external trappings of the glorified Virgin; but of course the Calvinist Spenser
cannot identify the Virgin, mother only of the
body of Christ, as

> The soveraine dearling of the Deity.[1]

In 1655 Thomas Stanley translated for his
History of Philosophy Benivieni's *Ode*, and selec-
tions from Pico's commentary. Stanley's translation, in octosyllabic couplets, is fluent and easy,
but hardly attempts to render the subtler meanings of the original.

[1] Fuller proofs of this interpretation of the *Fowre Hymnes*
I have developed elsewhere, but not at present in print.

ODE OF LOVE

Composed by Jerome Benivieni, Florentine Citizen, according to the Mind and Opinion of Platonists

STANZA I

Amor, dalle cui man sospes' el freno

Love, from whose hands suspended hang the reins

Del mio cor pende, et nel cui sacro regno

Unto my heart, who in his high empire

Nutrir non hebbe ad sdegno

Scorns not to feed the fire

La fiamma che per lui già in quel fu accesa,

By him enkindled in me long ago,

Muove la lingua mia, sforza, l' ingegno

Would move my tongue, my faculties inspire

Ad dir di lui quel che l' ardente seno

To tell what my enamored breast retains 6

Chiude; ma il cor vien meno,

Of him; but courage wanes;

Et la lingua repugna à tanta impresa,

My tongue to utter such high things is slow,

1–8. The poet is given the impulse and the inspiration to reveal the nature of Intellectual Love, by which all his desires are governed, of which his soul has reminiscence, and to which he evermore aspires.

Cf. Spenser, *Hymne in Honour of Love*, ll. 1–7, 15–21. Also *Hymne of Heavenly Beautie*, ll. 6–7.

Ne quel ch' en me può
   dir ne far difesa;
Et pur convien che' l
   mio concetto esprima
Forza contro ad mag-
   gior forza non vale.

Balks at the burden, nor
   excuse can show;
And yet my message it
   must needs impart,
Strength against great-
   er strength availing
   nought. 11

Ma perchè al pigro in-
   gegno amor quell' ale

Since Love has prom-
   ised to my sluggish
   thought

Promesso ha, con le
   qual nel cor mio in
   prima
Discese, benchè in cima
Credo per mai partir
   dalle sue piume

Those wings wherewith
   he entered first my
   breast,
Therein on high to nest,
And thence, methinks,
   now never to take
   flight; 15

Fa nido, quanto el lume
Del suo vivo splendor
   fia al cor mio scorta
Spero aprir quel che
   di lui ascoso hor
   porta.

So in the guiding light
Of his live glory I may
   still disclose
What of him privily my
   spirit knows.

12–18. Love condescending to the soul, by the same act draws the soul upward to itself. The object of Intellectual Love is Absolute Truth, to which, so far as he is able to follow Love's leading, the poet may attain.

14. *On high.* To indicate the higher, or intellectual, faculties.

Stanza II

Io dico com' amor dal divin fonte
Dell' increato ben qua giù s' infonde;
Quando in pria nato, et donde,
Muov' el ciel, l' alme informa, e' l mondo regge;
Come poi ch' entro alli human cor s' asconde,
Con qual et quanto al ferir dextr' et promte
Armi, è levar la fronte
Da terra sforz' al ciel l' humana gregge;

Com' arda, infiammi, advampi; e con qual legge
Quest' al ciel volga, et quello ad terra hor pieghi

I tell how Love from its celestial source
In Primal Good flows to the world of sense;
When it had birth; and whence; 21
How moves the heavens, refines the soul, gives laws
To all; in men's hearts taking residence,
With what arms keen and ready in resource,
It is the gracious force
Which mortal minds from earth to heaven draws; 26
How it may light, warm, burn; and what the cause
One love may earthward bend, one heavenward bear,

19–26. The poet will follow in his exposition the descent of Love from God through various intermediaries to the human soul, and then retrace its ascent back again to God by several grades.

Hor infra questi dua
l' inclini et fermi.

A third sustain mid-
way 'twixt earth and
heaven.   29

Stanche mie rime e voi
languidi e 'nfirmi.

My feeble rhymes, and
ye lame and uneven

Versi, hor ch' en terra
sia che per voi
preghi !

Verses, for you may
there be some to care,

Sì che à più giusti
prieghi

So that to worthier
prayer

Del' infiammato cor
s' inclin' Apollo;

Of kindled heart Apollo
may incline ;

Troppo aspro giogo el
collo

Too heavy for neck of
mine

Preme : Amor, le pro-
messe penne hor porgi

The yoke : O Love,
on my weak wings
now plight   35

27-28. *Carnal love*, which we share with the brutes ; *intellectual love*, which we may share with the Angels ; *human
love*, which is a mixture of carnal and intellectual love.

33. *Apollo.* The poet has already invoked Love to be
his guide : through loving he will have intelligence of Love.
He invokes Apollo that he may express this intelligence with
eloquence.

Cf. Spenser, *Hymne in Honour of Love*, ll. 22-28.   Cf. l. 24
and Benivieni, ll. 55-56 : —

Where thou doest sit in Venus
lap above.

Questi perchè nell' amorose
braccia
Della bella Cyprigna in
prima nacque.

All' ale 'nferme, e il
    camin cieco scorgi !

The promised pinions,
    and the blind way
    light !

STANZA III

Quando dal vero ciel
    converso, scende

When from true heaven
    deflected, radiance
    flows

Nell' angelica mente el
    divin sole,

To mind angelic from
    the highest sun,

Che la sua prima prole

And on that first-born
    one

Sotto le vive frondi
    illustra e' nforma, —

Pours light and form
    through living leaves
    defined, —   40

Stanza III. How love is awakened in the spirit of the first created Angel by contemplation of the celestial Venus, that is to say, of the Ideas emanating from the One Truth, which is God.

37–40. The angelic mind is the first emanation from God, or perfect Unity; this mind contains implicitly the archetypal Ideas, which are made explicit to it by the illumination of God's love and the ever growing desire for self-explication kindled and fed by that illumination.

37. *True heaven.* The perfect unity of God, in and for itself.

38. *Highest sun.* God.

40. *Through living leaves.* According to Diotima, in Plato's *Symposium*, Love was born in the Garden of Jove, on Venus's birthday, of Poros (Wealth) and Penia (Want). "The Garden of Jove," explains Ficino (*In convivium Platonis de amore*

Lei, ch' el suo primo
    ben ricerca et vuole
Per innato disio che
    quell' accende,
In lui reflessa prende
Virtù che 'l ricco sen
    depinge et forma.

Quinc' el primo disio che
    lei trasforma
Al vivo sol dell' incre-
    ato luce
Mirabilmente alhor s'
    incende e 'nfiamma.

This, that its first good
    longs to look upon
By natural desire which
    for that glows,
To that, reflected, owes
Power to express the
    wealth   in   itself
    shrined.

Then is the first desire
    which turns the mind
To the living sun of
    uncreated light   46
More wondrously in-
    flamed and set on
    fire.

commentarium, *Orat.* VI, *cap.* vii), "signifies the fecundity
of the angelic essence, in which, when there descends Poros,
that is to say the radiance of God, to union with Penia, that
is to say the Want which has been before in the Angel, Love
is born." Following out the figure of the Garden, Benivieni
means by "living leaves" the archetypal Ideas themselves,
which, fostered by Love, are conceived as growing out of the
angelic mind itself.

42. *Natural (innato) desire.* Before the mind is illuminated, before, so to speak, it is self-conscious, the desire which
is to govern its whole being, is only potential; yet once it is
called into actuality, it is recognized as natural, and no mere
accident.

45. *Lures the mind.* The desire of the lover is to become
one with the beloved. The ideal aspiration of the Angelic
mind is to become one with God, that is, to attain to the Idea
of its Ideas, the Unity behind its Diversity.

Quell' ardor, quell' incendio, et quella fiamma,	That heat, that glow, that flaming of desire,
Che dalla oscura mente et dalla luce	Which, in the mind obscure by heavenly light
Presa dal ciel, reluce	Kindled, now makes so bright 50
Nella angelica mente, è 'l primo et vero	The mind angelic, is the first and true
Amor, pio desidero	Love, the devotion due
D' inopia nato et di richezza alhora	Born then of want and wealth when of the skies
Che di se il ciel facea, chi Cypri honora.	She was conceived, whom Cyprus glorifies.

49. *Mind obscure.* Cf. notes above, ll. 40, 42. The dark mind, in which Ideas are still implicit only, is the Want (l. 53); the heavenly light is the Wealth (l. 53), of which Love is born.

53–54. Love and Beauty (Venus) the object of love, must be born at one and the same time, since they imply one another; yet since Beauty (Venus) occasions Love, Venus is described not only as older, but as the mother of Love.

48–52. Cf. Spenser, *Hymne in Honour of Love*, 64–65.

52–54. Cf. *ib.* 50–54.

The *prima prole*, or *angelica mente*, or Logos, Spenser in the *Hymne of Heavenly Love* (ll. 29–35) identifies, after St. John, with Christ, God's "eldest sonne and heire" and "firstling of his joy." The Holy Ghost, or

Stanza IV

Questi perchè nell' am- orose braccia	This Love, for that he on the amorous breast 55
Della bella Cyprigna in prima nacque,	Of the fair Cyprian at the first has lain,

that third from them derived,
Most wise, most holy, most almightie Spright,

(*Ib.* ll. 38–39.)

is the Christianized equivalent of Benivieni's alma (l. 75). In the *Hymne of Heavenly Beautie*, "Sapience," the Wisdom of the Angelic Mind, is identified at once with the celestial Venus, and with the Holy Ghost. Ficino had already indicated the former identification. "Since," he says,[1] "the Angelic Mind has being, life, and intelligence, they [the platonists] call its Being, or Essence, Saturn; its Life, Jove; its Intelligence, Venus." The analogy with the Christian Trinity is obvious.

The *vero ciel* (l. 37) is indicated by Spenser in the *Hymne of Heavenly Love*, ll. 57–60 —

the heavens illimitable hight
(Not this round heaven, which we from hence behold,
Adornd with thousand lamps of burning light,
And with ten thousand gemmes of shyning gold, etc.)

Stanza IV. Properties and effects of Intellectual, or Heavenly, Love: how the Ideal Beauty (celestial Venus), emanating from God, irradiates Material Beauty (terrestrial Venus), and how each evokes a corresponding love.

55–63. As Intellectual Love pursuing Intelligible Beauty (of the Ideas), aspires to God, so Human Love also by rising to Intellectual Love.

[1] *Comm. Sympos. Platon.*, II, vii.

Sempre seguir li piacque	To follow still is fain
L' ardente sol di sua bellezza viva.	The starry splendor of her fairest face.
Quinc' el primo disio che 'n noi si giacque	Hence our first stirrings of desire attain
Per lui di nuova canapè s'allaccia,	Through him an object newly manifest; 60
Che l' honorata traccia	And sharing his high quest,
Di lui seguendo, al primo ben n' adriva.	The way to highest good we too retrace.
Da lui el foco, per cui da lui deriva	By him the fire through which his living grace
Ciò ch' en lui vive, in noi s' accende, etdove	Distils, in us is lit; in flames whereof
Arde morendo el cor, ardendo cresce.	The heart consuming dies, yet dying lives.
Per lui el fonte immortal trabocca, ond' esce	Through him pours the live fountain, whence derives 66

65. As the perfection of Intellectual Love is the extinction of Sensual Love, so to live in the spirit we die in the flesh.

66–67. Love is the agency through which God creates and moves the physical universe.

70–72. Intellectual Love illuminates our ideas, shadows of the archetypal Ideas, until, the realities taking the place of their shadows, our love becomes as the love of angels, who are illuminated directly by God.

55–58. Cf. Spenser, *Hymne in Honour of Love*, 61–62; 71–73.

Ciò che poi el ciel qua giù formando move.	What heaven then shaping here below does move.
Da lui converse piove	Diffused is through this Love
Quel lume in noi che sopr' à ciel ci tira. In noi per lui respira	That light in us which leads us to the skies. Through him within us rise 70
Quel increato sol tanto splendore Che l' alma infiamma in noi d' eterno amore.	Splendors reflected from the sun supernal Until our souls are lit with love eternal.

STANZA V

Come del primo ben l' eterna mente È, vive, intende, intende, muove, e finge	As from first good the eternal intelligence Is, lives, conceives, so conceives, moves, creates

66–67. *Ib.* 74–75.

59–62.⎫
68–72.⎭ *Ib.* 106–109.

Stanza V. How the World-Soul, by participation in the Ideas of the Intelligible World (the eternal Intelligence) creates the Sensible Universe, reflecting upon it the shadow of the divine Beauty (Earthly Venus), which is the object of Sensual Love.

K

L' alma; spiega e depinge
Per lei quel sol ch' illustra 'l divin petto:

Quinci ciò ch' el pio sen concepe et stringe,

Diffunde; et ciò che poi si muove et sente,

Per lei mirabilmente

Mosso, sente, vive, opra ogni suo effetto.
Da lei, come dal ciel nell' intelletto,

The soul; where germinates   75
Each living ray shed from the breast divine,
Till from the soul's meek brooding emanates
That which endowed with motion then and sense,
Through the soul's influence,
Lives, feels, fulfilling each innate design.
And from that soul, as the heavenly from God's shrine,   81

73–75. The archetypal Ideas derive from First Good (*i.e.* God); the Angelic Mind receives them as they are in themselves *sub specie æternitatis;* the Rational Soul receives them *sub specie temporis* from the Angelic Mind. The Mind therefore is contemplative, or static; the Soul active, or dynamic, the Mind *is,* the Soul *becomes.* From the Soul (ὁ δημιουργός), then, proceeds that which becomes, that is to say, the physical universe, endowed with motion and sense.

75–80. As the Rational Soul reproduces after her fashion the Ideas reflected in her by the Mind, so the Sensitive Soul expresses, as fully as Matter allows, these reflected Ideas in the physical universe.

81–83. As divine, or intellectual, Beauty is the reflection

Nasce Vener qua giù,
  la cui bellezza
Splende in ciel, vive in
  terra, el mondo adom-
  bra.
L' altra, che dentr' al sol
  si specchia all' ombra

Di quel ch'al contem-
  plar per lei s' advezza,
Com' ogni sua richezza

Prende dal vivo sol
  ch' en lei refulge,
Così sua luce indulge

Is earthly Venus born,
  whose beauty lights
The skies, inhabits
  earth, is nature's veil.

The heavenly, who from
  the sun is mirrored
  pale
Within his shade whose
  musing she incites,
As she receives her
  lights 86
Ev'n from the living
  sun that in her glows,
So she her light bestows

of God, the Idea of Ideas, in the Mind; so earthly, or sensible, Beauty, is the reflection in the sensitive Soul of God also, but as refracted through the interposed media of Mind and Rational Soul.

84–85. Heavenly Beauty, or Venus, is visible to those who in contemplation seek her, but as through the glass, darkly, of their mortality.

86–89. Cf. note to ll. 81–83.

89, 90. *Love profane*, limited to the senses, cannot reach beyond sensible Beauty.

78–90. Cf. Spenser, *Hymne in Honour of Beautie*, ll. 29 ff.
What time this world's great
  workmaister (*i.e.*, the Dem-
  iurge, or Rational Soul) did
  cast
To make al things such as we
  now behold,

A questa; et come amor celeste in lei

On the earthly; and while sacred love is hers,

Pende, così el volgar segue costei.

To her base sister love profane defers. 90

It seemes that he before his eyes had plast
A goodly paterne, etc. (*i.e.*, the Ideas of *l'eterna mente*).
That wondrous paterne, wheresoere it bee,
Whether in earth layd up in secret store,
Or else in heaven . . .
Is perfect Beautie which all men adore, etc.
. . . through infusion of celestiall powre
The duller earth it quickneth with delight
And life-full spirits privily doth powre
Through all the parts, that to the lookers sight
They seem to please. That is thy soveraine might,
O Cyprian queene, which, flowing from the beame
Of thy bright starre, thou into them doest streame . . .
Thence to the soule darts amorous desyre, etc.

(L' altra, che dentr 'al sol, si specchia all' ombra.
Di quel ch' al contemplar per lei s' advezza.)

(. . . ciò che poi si muove et sente
Par lei mirabilmente

Mosso, sente, vive, opra ogni suo effetto.)

(Com' ogni sua richezza

Prende dal vivo sol ch'en lei refulge,
Così sua, luce indulge etc.)

As Benivieni in ll. 89–90 distinguishes between sacred and profane love according to the two kinds of Beauty, so Spenser at large in ll. 64 ff.

Stanza VI

Quando formata, in pria dal divin volto	Whenas full-formed, first from the countenance blest
Per descendere qua giù l' alma si parte,	Down hither to descend the soul departs,
Dalla più eccelsa parte	It from the highest parts
Ch' alberghi el sol nel cor human s' imprime	That lodge the sun to man's heart takes its way
Dov' esprimendo con mirabil arte	Wherein applying with consummate arts 95

Stanza VI. How, descending into the human heart, the Rational Soul shapes the body, so far as the body's particular material make-up permits, in accordance with her heavenly lights, that is to say, the Ideas in which she participates, modified by the influence of the planet under which the individual was born; and how the resulting beauty of that body, seen by another person, born under a like influence of the planets, awakens love in the soul of that person, whose enamoured Imagination then transfigures the image of the beloved one with new and greater beauty.

95–98. The Soul, incarnated, has still reminiscence of her *wealth, erstwhile celestial*, the archetypal Ideas, and after their model she strives to shape the body she inhabits. At the same time she is directly influenced by the planets: thus an individual born under Jove will have a "jovial" temperament, one under Saturn a "saturnine," one under Mercury a "mercurial," etc. From the planets, accordingly, proceeds the

Quel valor poi che da
sua stella ha tolto,
Et che nel grembo ac-
colto
Vive di sue celeste spo-
glie prime, —
Quanto nel seme human
posson sue lime,
Forma suo albergo; in
quel fabrica et stampa
C' hor più hor men re-
pugna al divin culto.

Indi qual' hor dal sol
ch' en lei ne sculto

Virtue whereof 'tis from
its star possessed,
And bearing in its breast

Models erstwhile celes-
tial, — well as may
Avail its tools, it builds
of human clay
Its house, molding
such matter into form
As thwarts now less
now more its high
designs.   101
And sometimes will the
sun   that   therein
shines

differentiation of incarnated souls by temperamental types.
Further differentiation — sex, character, personal appearance,
etc. — is caused by the infinite varieties in the composition
of the material elements of the body itself, always therefore
more or less irreducible to the ideal types registered in the
formative Soul.

105–108. See notes to Stanza VI. In ll. 102–117 Benivieni traces rapidly and generally the reascent of the Soul
guided by Love. After this general sketch, he rebegins the
ascent, grade by grade, with l. 117. Stanzas VI, VII, and
VIII thus overlap in idea, and form one whole. Pico suggests
that the whole poem has thus six parts corresponding in number to the six grades of ascent, and further that the overlapping
of stanzas VI, VII, and VIII symbolizes the impropriety of
stopping the Soul on its upward way.

Scende nell' altrui cor
   l' infusa stampa;
Se gli è conforme, ad-
   vampa
L' alma; qual poi ch' en
   se l' alberga assai

Stamp on another heart
   the imprinted form;
Which, meetly matched,
   will warm
That soul; and lodg-
   ing there will erelong
   blaze   105

91–100. Cf. Spenser, *Hymne in Honour of Beautie*, ll. 106–119:

> For when the soule, the which derived was,
> At first, out of that great immortal Spright,
> By whom all live to love, whilome did pas
> Downe from the top of purest heavens light,
> To be embodied here, it then tooke light
> And lively spirits from that fairest starre,
> Which lights the world forth from his firie carre.
>
> Which powre retayning still, or more or less,
> When she in fleshly seede is oft enraced,
>   (Benivieni: *nel seme human.*)
> Through every part she doth the same impresse,
> According as the heavens have her raced,
> And frames her house, in which she will be placed,
> Fit for her selfe, adorning it with spoyle
> Of th' heavenly riches which she robd erewhyle.
>   (Benivieni: *sua celeste spoglie prime.*)

100–101. Spenser, *ib.* 124–126, 141–147: —

> And the grosse matter by a soveraine might
> Tempers so trim, that it may well be seene
> A pallace fit for such a virgin queene.
>   *   *   *   *   *   *
> Yet oft it falles that many a gentle mynde
> Dwels in deformed tabernacle drownd,

Più bella à divin rai	Far fairer in the rays
Di sua virtù l'effinge :	Of that soul's virtue :
et di qui nasce	whence is it decreed
Ch' amando el cor d' un	That loving hearts on
dolce error si pasce.	a sweet error feed.

> Either by chaunce, against the course of kynd,
> Or through unaptnesse in the substance fownd,
> Which it assumed of some stubborne grownd,
> That will not yield unto her formes direction,
>   (Benivieni : *repugna al divin culto.*)
> But is deform'd with some foule imperfection.

Pico begins his commentary on Stanza VI with an *excursus* (after Ficino) on the nature of Beauty, which, he argues, does not consist in "the material disposition of the body," its proportions and coloring, but on a certain spiritual quality of "grace." Spenser develops the same view in ll. 57 ff. Later in his commentary on this stanza, Pico declaims against lust of fleshly Beauty; Spenser incorporates a similar sermon in ll. 148–174.

102–105. Cf. Spenser, *ib.* 175–210 (I quote only the more relevant lines).

> Therefore, to make your beauty more appeare,
> It you behoves to love, and forth to lay
> That heavenly riches which in you ye bears,
> That men the more admyre their fountaine may ;
> For else what booteth that celestial ray,
> If it in darkness be enshrined ever,
> That it of loving eyes be vewed never ?
>
> * * * * * *
>
> But in your choice of loves, this well advize,
> That likest to your selves ye them select,
> The which your forms first source may sympathize. . . .
>
> * * * * * *

Stanza VII

Pascesi el cor d' un dolce error, l' amato	On a sweet error the heart feeds, its dear
Obietto in se come in sua prole guardando,	One deeming that which of itself was born ; 110
	Grade II–III.
Talhor poi reformando Quell' al lume divin che 'n lui n' impresso,	May this then readorn With light divine whereof it is possessed —
	Grade IV.
Raro e celeste don, quinc' elevando	A rare, high gift ! — and still thus upward borne,
Di grado in grado se nell' increato	May grade by grade to the uncreated sphere Grade V.
Sol torna, ond' è formato	Return, whence fashioned were 115

For love is a celestiall harmonie
Of likely harts composed of starres concent.
Cf. also *Hymne in Honour of Love*, ll. 120–124.

105–108. Spenser does not, like Benivieni, go twice over the grades of the purification of love. It is more convenient, therefore, to cite the parallels to these lines in connection with the next stanza.

Stanza VII. The reascent of the Soul. After a preliminary and summary outline of the Soul's ascent (ll. 102–117), Benivieni restates the threefold source of Beauty, and then retraces, grade by grade, the Soul's progress, under Love's guidance, from lowest to highest Beauty.

Ne quel che nell' amato
obietto è' spresso.

All beauties in the loved
one manifest.

Grade VI.

Per tre fulgidi specchi
un sol da esso

One sun enkindles from
that countenance
blest

Volto divin raccende
ogni beltate

Through three refulgent
glasses every grace

Che la mente, lo spirto,
e' l corpo adorna.

That mind and soul and
body here adorns.

Quinci gli occhi, et per
gli occh' ove soggiorna

Thus first the eyes, next
through these whence
sojourns   120

117–119. The one glory of God, variously reflected and refracted through the Angelic nature, or Intelligible World, the Rational nature, or Spiritual World, the Corporeal nature, or Sensible World, is the source of beauty in the human mind and soul and body.

120–126. Grades I–III in the ascent of the Soul, supplementing ll. 102–110. Grade I — The heart embraces the fairness conveyed to it through the eyes, or outer sense; that is, the loved object is physical and external. Grade II — The heart embraces the fairness of the loved object as represented by *its other handmaid*, viz. the Imagination, or inner sense, which renders it, *though less base, not full* expressed; that is, the loved object becomes a glorified subjective image, fairer than reality and fully possessed by the lover. It is the *sweet error* of love that it thus in imagination sees the loved object fairer than it is — at least for others. Still, perfect beauty is not *full expressed* in this sensuous image, not even perfect sensuous beauty. The image, however glorified, is of a particular *fairness*, which only participates in, but does not

L' altra su' ancilla, el cor   Its other handmaid,
li spoglie ornate.   does the heart em-
                                                      brace

fully express, its perfect type: so, as the Greek painter is said
to have shaped his perfect type of beautiful woman by com-
bining in one the beauties of a hundred women, the Soul now
— Grade III — from many *fairs torn from matter*, *i.e.* from
many subjective images of particular fairness, forms the image,
still sensuous indeed, of the type. Continuing the process,
the Soul may reach to a conception embracing in one image,
at least symbolically, all sensible Beauty — as, to take a
modern illustration, Hogarth's "curve of beauty."

113. It is a *rare, high gift* that inspires the Soul to turn
aside wholly from the senses to contemplate the divinity
which resides in herself.

Stanzas VII and VIII are virtually telescoped by Spenser
into *Hymne in Honour of Beautie*, ll. 211–238, but his plan requires a return to the human plane of love: having climbed
with Benivieni the "ladder of love" to "heavenly beautie,"
he as a lover invests his lady with the radiance of that, thus
continuing to the end the "dolce error," which Benivieni's
"Soul" transcends. I quote Spenser's lines, indicating the
closer parallels, though the parallelism of the general argument
is even more striking.

True lovers, *i.e.* those matched by their stars, behold each
other (*Hymne in Honour of Beautie*, l. 211): —

Drawing out of the object of   (*I.e.* Grade I — Benivieni,
  their eyes   102–105, 120.)
A more refined forme, which   (Grade II — *spoglia ornate
  they present   reformate*, 121–122.)
Unto their mind, voide of all   (Grade III — ll. 123–126.)
  blemishment;
Which it reducing to her first
  perfection,

Prend' in lei reformate,

Non però espresse; indi
di varie e molte
Beltà, dal corpo sciolte,

That fairness, though
less base,

Not full expressed; un-
til from many fairs
The heart from matter
tears,

Beholdeth free from fleshes
frayle infection.
And then conforming it unto
the light,
Which in it selfe it hath remaining still,
Of that first sunne, yet sparck-
ling in his sight,
Thereof he fashions in his
higher skill
An heavenly beautie to his
fancies will,
And it embracing in his mind
entyre,
The mirrour of his owne
thought doth admyre.

(Grade IV — ll. 111–112. —
Talhor poi reformando
Quell' al lume divin che' n lui
n' impresso. . . .)

(ll. 131–134.)

(Grade V — ll. 138–139. —
Quinci, mentr' el pio cor
l' alme vestige
Segue, entro alla sua ment'
el ved' inserto.)

Which seeing now so inly
faire to be,

As outward it appeareth to
the eye,
And with his spirits propor-
tion to agree,
He thereon fixeth all his fan-
tasie,

(ll. 127–128. —
Quinc' Amor l' alm' in quest,
e 'l cor deletta ;

In lui, com' in suo parto, anchor vaneggia.)

Form' un concetto, in
  çui quel che natura
Divis' ha in tutti, in un
  pinge e figura.

Is shaped a type, where-
  in what nature rends
In all asunder, into one
  image blends.   126

Stanza VIII

Quinc' amor l' alm' in
  quest' e 'l cor de-
  letta ;

Thus by this type love
  heart and soul de-
  lights ;

Counting it fairer than it is
  indeede,

And yet indeede her faire-
  nesse doth exceede.
For lovers' eyes more sharply
  sighted bee
Than other mens. . . .

(ll.   129–130. — Che men-
    tre el ver vaneggia,
Come raggio di sol sott' acqu'
  el vede.)

(l.   108. — . . . amando el
    cor d' un dolce error si
    pasce.)

Cf. *Hymne in Honour of Love*, ll. 190 ff.

Stanza VIII. As in Grade II the *sweet error* of the enamoured Heart was to identify the glorified image created by the
Imagination with the external object of desire, so now in
Grade III the Soul rejoices in the universalized conception
of sensible Beauty, still believing the principle of Beauty
therein contained to be given her from the Sensible World.
But reflecting on this principle, the Soul discovers that the
Sensible World has given but the raw material, and that the
principle itself of Beauty is of her own making, and is only the
reflection of the divine Ideas as conceived by her. Her loved
object, therefore, — Grade IV, — wholly withdrawn from
Sense, is manifested in her own proper Ideal, namely, Spiritual
Beauty or the *Moral* Ideals of Justice, Courage, and Temperance (ll. 131–137). But these Moral Ideals, appropriate

In lui, com' in suo parto,
anchor vaneggia,

On this, as on their off-
spring, still they
smile;

Che, mentre el ver va-
gheggia,

Where long-sought
truth the while

Come raggio di sol sott'
acqu' el vede.

Is as a sun-ray under
water seen. 130

Pur non so che divin
ch' en lui lampeggia,

For in that imaged fair-
ness glimmers still,

Benchè adumbrat', el
cor pietoso allecta

Though darkly, some-
thing sacred that in-
vites

Da questa ad più per-
fecta

The gentle heart to
heights

to the Soul as *active*, themselves imply standards beyond the
sphere of action, namely the intellectual Ideals of Wisdom,
Knowledge, and Judgment. Therefore, — Grade V, — the
Soul turns now (ll. 138–139) from action to thought: the
loved object is found in the Mind. But the individual Mind,
thinking discursively from premise to premise, implies in the
last analysis major premises that are not deduced by the
Mind itself, but are axiomatic truths, — truths, in other words,
that the individual Mind does not reason out but intuit.
Thus — Grade VI (ll. 140–144) — the Soul in her pilgrimage
is led above and beyond the Individual Mind to the intuition
of eternal and universal Ideas whose seat is in the Eternal
and Universal, or Angelic Mind, the Intelligible World.

129–130. The spiritual principle of Beauty is still darkened
by the sensible image in which it is represented as a ray of
sun is darkened by the water into which it shines.

133. *Heights*. The rational as opposed to the sensitive
activity of the Soul.

Beltà, ch' en cima à
   quel superba siede.
Ivi non l' ombra pur
   ch' en terra fede

Del vero ben ne dia
   scorge, ma certo

Lume e del vero sol
   più ver' effige.
Quinci mentr' el pio cor
   l' alme vestige
Segue, entro alla sua
   ment' el ved' inserto ;
Inde à più chiaro et
   aperto
Lum' appresso ad quel
   sol sospeso vola,
Dalla cui viva et sola
Luce informat' amando
   si fa bello

Where a more perfect
   beauty sits serene.
There not the shadow
   that on earth has
   been   135
Sole witness of true
   good, the heart shall
   find,
But clear light and the
   true sun's image true.
If gentle heart those
   sacred signs pursue,
It finds that image
   planted in the mind ;
Thence soars to more
   refined   140
And pure light circum-
   fused about that sun
By whose eternal, one
Glory illumined, lov-
   ing, are made fair

135–136. Sensible Beauty is only the *shadow* of *true good*, or *Divine* Beauty ; but the shadow is the only earthly witness of that, as the Love it excites is the only earthly impulse which leads the Soul upwards.

137. *Image true.* The Soul's Moral Beauty faithfully embodies true Beauty, but in the sphere of action, or "becoming," which is lower than the sphere of contemplation, or "being."

142–144. Cf. 117–119.

La mente, l' alma, e' l mondo et ciò ch' è 'n quello.	The mind, the soul, the world, and all things there.

In the *Hymne in Honour of Beautie*, Spenser rises only to Grade V — Intellectual Beauty as seen by the Individual Mind, *i.e.* Truth or Sapience *sub specie temporis* — but in the *Hymne of Heavenly Beautie*, he discusses, without reverting to the lower grades, Grade VI — Intellectual Beauty, or Sapience in itself, *sub specie eternitatis*. Above the visible heavens, he says, are others "unmoving, uncorrupt" (ll. 64 ff.), where dwell the

... pure Intelligences from God inspired,

i.e. Benivieni's "angelica mente." Above these is God, who is the Unity from which they proceed, but more than their sum: —

Yet is that Highest farre beyond all telling,
Fairer than all the rest which there appeare,
Though all their beauties joynd together were.
(ll. 101–103.)

God's "perfectnesse," however,

... unto all he daily doth display,

(Cf. Benivieni, ll. 117–119: —
Per tre fulgidi specchi un sol da esso

And shew himselfe in the image of his grace,

Volto divin raccendo ogni beltate

As in a looking glasse.
(ll. 113–115.)

Che la mente, lo spirto, e'l corpo adorna.)

To this divine Beauty, the mind may mount through heavenly contemplation (ll. 134 ff.). Cf. Benivieni, ll. 141–144. And Spenser concludes by painting this divine, or Intellectual, Beauty as "Sapience," declaring of her, as Benivieni of the celestial Venus: —

STANZA IX

Canzon, io sente Amor	O song of mine, I feel
ch' el fren raccoglie	Love drawing rein
Al temerario ardir ch'el	On the rash ardors that
cor mio sprona	my spirit move 146
Frose di là dal desti-	Beyond the path ap-
nato corso :	pointed to aspire :
Rafrena el van disio,	He applies the curb ;
restring' el morso.	he checks the vain
	desire.

Both heaven and earth obey unto her will,
And all the creatures which they both containe.
> (ll. 197–198.)

Contemplation of her is the "sabbath" of the Soul, as Pico calls it, when, in Spenser's words (l. 301) : —

Thy straying thoughts henceforth for ever rest.

Stanza IX. 145–148. The Intelligible World of Ideas, to which the desirous Soul has by intuition risen, is itself not the *full expression* (cf. l. 123) of Ideal Beauty. The eternal and universal Ideas which constitute and form it, form together the Absolute Truth in itself, but in their self-consciousness; the Universal, or Angelic, Mind, they appear not as One, but as Many. Their Unity, or "togetherness," is God ; and God, as perfect Unity, cannot be self-conscious, since this, distinguishing itself as subject and object, is *ipso facto*, a violation of Unity. While there is self-consciousness, therefore, union of the Soul with God Himself is unattainable. Plotinus, indeed, and other mystics have found in Ecstasy a state of the Soul in which self-consciousness is lost, a possibility of such union even during this life ; but from consideration of that "Sabbath" of the Soul, Benivieni abstains ; enough to consider her "six days' labor."

L

Etcasti orechi à quel ch' amor ragiona	And now, chaste ears to all that speak of love
Hor volgi; se persona	Turn thou; and if there prove 150
Truovi che dal tu' amor s' inform' et vesta,	One with thy love informed and garmented,
Non pur le frondi à questa	Before him do not spread
Del tuo divin thesor, ma 'l frutto spiega;	Thy garner's frondage only, but its fruit;
Agli altri basti l' un, ma l' altro niega.	The first alone vouchsafe to other suit.

153–154. Cf. Dante (Canz. *Voi che intendendo.* Envoy.)

> O song of mine, methinks they shall be rare
> Who may thee rightly understand in all,
> So intricate and subtle is thy skill:
> Wherefore if peradventure it befall
> That thou in presence of such folk shalt fare
> As seem to understand thy meaning ill,
> I pray thee then that thou take comfort still,
> Saying, my youngest well-beloved, to them:
> "Observe, at least, how beautiful I am."

DID "ASTROPHEL" LOVE "STELLA"?

In 1591, the sonnet-sequence by Sir Philip Sidney, entitled *Astrophel and Stella* was produced surreptitiously by the publisher, Thomas Newman. Of the numerous interesting questions concerning these ostensible love-sonnets, the one I wish here to raise — or raise again, for it is an old one — is the question of their personal sincerity. Did "Astrophel" love "Stella"?

In general, I am not partial to this type of literary question. There is much in Browning's contention that the poet's self, his "house of life," is his castle, not penetrable by right or power of any gossip-mongering critic. To that class he replies scornfully, "You can't get in anyway!"

> whoso desires to penetrate
> Deeper, must dive by the spirit-sense —
> No optics like yours, at any rate!

But it is hard for an ordinary human being not to ask after any story, "Is it really true?" And the world at large is credulous, inclining to take people

147

— even poets — at their word. Heine certainly
gave a most undeserved compliment, when he
said —

> Diese Welt glaubt nicht an Flammen,
> Und sie nimmt's für Poesie.

On the contrary, the world, — at least the biog-
raphers, critics, and schoolgirls, — dubious about
Poesie, has calmly taken it all for *Flammen*,
forgetting old Giles Fletcher's prudent consideration that "a man may write of love and not be in
love; as well as of husbandry and not go to the
plough; or of witches and be none; or of holiness and be flat profane." [1] Are we to believe
Sidney, or not, when he protests —

> know! that I, in pure simplicity,
> Breathe out the flames which burn within my heart,
> Love only reading unto me this art.   — xxviii.

Are we to believe Dante, or not, when he protests
so similarly —

> Io mi son un che, quando
> Amor mi spira, noto, ed a quel modo
> Che detta dentro, vo significando.
> > *Purgatorio*, xxiv, 52–54.

Certainly, what each says is *Poesie;* but is it
Flammen? While there is imagination, there is

[1] *Licia* (1593), Epist. Ded.

doubt. Coleridge may be right; a poet may be a poet just because he can compel us — nay, fool us — into "a willing suspension of disbelief" in his sincerity. A feigned artlessness, the profession of "pure simplicity," so far from reassuring, should give pause. Bret Harte's Heathen Chinee was most artless and simple.

So, if "pure simplicity" is a device within the capacity of the most ordinary actor, to convey the illusion of an overmastering passion is the triumph of a great artist. No one would deny this proposition in the abstract; yet how many critics have spun out heated arguments upon an implied denial! Listen to Swinburne defending the "sincerity" of Shakspere's Sonnets; or to coolerheaded Jusserand answering, only yesterday, my own titular question: "Like most of the poets of his time, Sidney *could* draw love songs from his imagination; he has strewn his prose 'Arcadia' with such. No one can read them without noticing the difference, and without concluding that, in truth, Astrophel loved Stella" (*Lit. Hist. Eng. People*, II [1906], 396, 397). By the same token, if poetic quality be the test of literal reality, then Juliet's love must be the reality and Shakspere's own "Will" sonnets to the Dark Lady the fiction, "for no one can read them without noticing the difference, and without concluding that, in truth,"

Juliet really lived and loved Romeo, and Shakspere — after such bad and plagiaristic puns —
could never have loved the Dark Lady!

Another up-to-date critic, Mr. Sidney Lee, reads
Sidney's sonnets, and concludes quite differently
from M. Jusserand.

> Although it is probable [he writes (*Eliz. Sonnets*,
> Introd. xliii)] that Sidney's pursuit of the favour of
> Lady Rich, a coquettish friend of his youth who mar-
> ried another, led him to turn sonneteer, the imitative
> quality that . . . is visible throughout Sidney's ample
> effort, . . . destroys most of those specious preten-
> sions to autobiographic confessions which the unwary
> reader may discern in them.

But, one may ask, does the "imitative quality"
of Milton's tender sonnet to his dead wife —
following as it does in its conception a similar
sonnet by Bernardino Rota ("In lieto, e pien di
reverenzia aspetto") — make its autobiographic
pretensions specious? or, more broadly, may not
a man go a-wooing or a-mourning as well in a
borrowed song as in a borrowed suit?

Thus from internal evidence, these two representative critics — and I take them simply as
representative — deduce opposite, and as I believe unnecessary, conclusions from the same
premises. External evidence likewise reads double
to them.

Sidney's poetic worship of Stella [comments Mr.
Lee (*loc. cit.*)] became a conventional theme in Elizabethan poetry, and enjoyed a popularity only second
to that of Petrarch's poetic worship of Laura. The
locus classicus for its treatment is the collection of elegies,
entitled *Astrophel*, to which Spenser was the chief con-
tributor. That volume was dedicated to Sidney's
widow, and his sister, the Countess of Pembroke, wrote
a poem for it. Throughout the work, Sidney's celebration of Stella is accounted his most glorious achieve-
ment in literature. The dedication of *Astrophel* to
Sidney's wife deprives of serious autobiographical
significance his description in the sonnets of his pursuit
of Stella's affections.

So Mr. Lee ; now M. Jusserand : —

Sidney's sonnets . . . came out . . . after his death ;
and the world knew then how deep had been the passion
that "Astrophel" had felt for "Stella." And Stella,
to the inconvenience of a very modern school of critics,
according to whom Sidney had described imaginary
loves, the true Stella, Penelope Devereux, Lady Rich,
in spite of her faults, more and more visible, in spite of
her far from exemplary life, remained, for the friends
of the Muses, a sacred and semi-divine being, for no
other reason than that she had been Sidney's love,
the subject of his verse. The opinion of contemporaries
is perhaps worth as much as that of the critics of three
hundred years later [*loc. cit.*].

Mr. Lee is speaking from the English point of
view; M. Jusserand from the French. It is

just barely possible — I will not emphasize the suggestion — that difference of nationality may to some degree account for their different way of taking, for instance, the so-called *locus classicus* of the celebration of Astrophel's pursuit of Stella, Spenser's elegy dedicated to Lady Essex, Sidney's widow that was. But had they examined the elegy itself more closely, they would have found in it, I think, means of reconcilement.

To begin with, Spenser's dedication was distinctly less to the widow of the dead Sidney than to the wife of the living Essex. The elegy, whenever written, was published in 1595, when Spenser was assiduously courting the patronage of Essex, just victorious at Cadiz, and now reigning favorite. Assuredly, Spenser would have taken no chances of wounding Lady Essex's sensibilities; and despite M. Jusserand's citation of the indulgence shown to Châteaubriand's outspokenness "concerning his own extremely real loves," I doubt if an Englishwoman would have welcomed even in those more "spacious days" the frank celebration of her late husband's infidelity, and her rival's triumph. Be that as it may, the apparently unregarded thing is that Spenser implies no marital infidelity, raises no question of real rivalry. Here is the gist of his indictment : —

> Stella the faire, the fairest star in skie,
> As faire as Venus or the fairest faire,

(A fairer star saw never living eie)
Shot her sharp pointed beames through purest aire.
  Her he did love, her he alone did honor,
  His thoughts, his rimes, his songs were all upon her.

To her he vowd the service of his daies,
  On her he spent the riches of his wit;
For her he made hymnes of immortall praise,
  Of onely her he sung, he thought, he writ. . . .

Ne her with ydle words alone he wowed,
  And verses vaine, (yet verses are not vaine)
But with brave deeds to her sole service vowed,
  And bold atchievements her did entertaine.

Undoubtedly, Spenser says that Astrophel
did love Stella — but *how?* was there not a
manner of loving recognized at the time as capable
of sincerity, even of fervency, and yet not in
wedlock, and still not illicit? Of course, every
one at all familiar with the Renaissance will
recognize that I mean platonic love. I have not
time here to discuss in detail the revival of
platonism, systematized as a scientific gospel in
the Florentine academy of Ficino and Pico della
Mirandola, and as a social gospel in the *Asolani* of
Bembo and the *Cortegiano* of Castiglione, and during the following century divulgated throughout
Europe. In the Renaissance and after, the social
gospel of platonic love was often treated with

levity or irony; but we cannot understand the
Renaissance, unless we remember that many
serious men and women took the notion seriously,
almost religiously. Castiglione, in fact, speaking
through Bembo, makes platonic love the virtual
religious basis of his ideal character, the power
in ourselves which makes for righteousness.
Moreover, platonic love was for him, and for others like him, more than a vague term for an honest
intimacy between men and women. It was a cult
with rules and limitations, duties and rewards,
as sharply defined as those of the medieval chivalric love-cult, from which, indeed, fused with
platonism proper, the Renaissance platonic love-
cult derived. Love is defined as desire awakened
by beauty, and by progressive illumination passes
from sensible beauty to spiritual, and from spiritual
beauty to divine — from lust to love, and from
love to religion. The duty of the lover is service
and honor — *prouesse* and *courtoisie* adapted to
the new social environment of the court; the
reward of the right lover is intellectual communion with his lady by conversation (*entrétiens du
cœur*) — "risi piacevoli, i ragionamenti domestici
e secreti, il motteggiare, scherzare, toccar la
mano" (Castiglione) — and supreme spiritual
communion in the kiss, the platonic sacrament;
for the kiss, says Castiglione, "is rather union of

soul than of body, since it has power to draw the
soul to itself, and separate it from the body"
("il bascio si pò più presto dir congiungimento
d' anima che di corpo, perchè in quella ha tanta
forza che la tira a sè, e la separa dal corpo").

Now in the light of this quintessential doctrine,
Spenser's account of Astrophel's "pursuit" of
Stella becomes quite different from the vulgar
liaison which shocks Mr. Lee, and is condoned
by M. Jusserand "quia poeta multum amavit,"
et bene dixit. Spenser's opening figure, the liken-
ing of Stella's influence to "beames" "shot"
from "fairest star in skie," recalls the most
exquisite epitome of platonic love in Michelangelo's

> Dalle più alte stelle
>   Discende uno splendore
>   Che 'l desir tira a quelle;
> E qui si chiama amore.

> (From highest stars above
>   Downward a radiance flows,
>   Drawing desire to those;
> And here men call it love.)

The rest is the declaration of Sidney's "service"
with "honor," in phrases virtually identical with
Spenser's own explicit utterance of platonism
in his *Hymne to Love* (especially vss. 204–224).
And in conformity with this interpretation of

Spenser's elegy is the testimony of Matthew
Roydon in the same series of elegies, that

> Above all others this (Sidney) is hee
> Which erst approoved in his song,
> That love and honour might agree,
> And that pure love will do no wrong.

Spenser and Roydon, at least, read Astrophel
and Stella as an expression ultimately of pure
platonic love, and so acclaimed it. Such love
was acceptedly licit toward a married woman;
indeed, in theory, it was most fitly so directed;
since the platonic, like the chivalric, love theorists
held that their union of pure spirit was incompatible with the grosser union of matrimony, especially as for the noble class primarily concerned
marriage was so largely a matter "of convenience."
There was accordingly no theoretically valid
reason for Lady Sidney to be jealous of Stella, or
for Lord Rich to be jealous of Astrophel, though
Sidney once or twice seems to imply that he was
(cf. xxiv, xxxvii, lxxviii).

But Castiglione, more practical-minded than
Bembo, made one prudent requirement for the
platonic lover: he must be no longer young.
Castiglione's ideal lovers were foreordained to be
Michelangelo at sixty-three "loving" Vittoria
Colonna at forty-eight. At the same time,
Castiglione will pardon the young passionate

lover, provided he will rise from the ashes of his dead passions to a higher love; and what Castiglione says on this point curiously fits Sidney's situation.

> . . . I believe that, although sensual love in every age of life is an evil (*malo*), yet in youths it is excusable, and even to some degree permissible (*licito*); for though it entails sufferings, perils, fatigues, and many unhappinesses, still there are many who to win the favor of loved ladies do excellent deeds, which although not directed to a good end, are yet in themselves good; and so from much bitterness extract a little sweetness, and through the adversities they endure recognize at last their error. . . . I pardon them their base love [he goes on] provided that in it they show gentleness (*gentilezza*), courtesy, and valor . . .; and when they are no longer of youthful age, they wholly abandon it, leaving that sensual desire, as the lowest rung of the ladder by which man climbs unto the true love.

At the beginning of the Sonnets, the young Sidney sees the better, yet cannot but follow the worse, love.

> It is most true — that eyes are formed to serve
> The inward light; and that the heavenly part
> Ought to be King; from whose rules, who doth swerve,
> (Rebels to Nature) strive for their own smart. . . .
> True — that true beauty, virtue is indeed;
> Whereof this beauty can be but a shade,
> Which elements with mortal mixture breed:
> True — that on earth, we are but pilgrims made;
> And should in soul, up to our country move:
> True — and yet true that I must Stella love. — v.

And his love, he admits, is not only thus imperfect, being of a mortal beauty (though participant in the immortal "elements"), but also his love is stained with passion.

> Alas! have I not pain enough? my friend!
> Upon whose breast, a fiercer gripe doth tire,
> Than did on him who first stole down the fire;
> While Love on me, doth all his quiver spend:
> But with your rhubarb words ye must contend
> To grieve me worse in saying, "That Desire
> Doth plunge my well-formed soul even in the mire
> Of sinful thoughts, which do in ruin end."

In the following sestette he protests indeed a pure love —

> If that be sin, which doth the manners frame
> Well stayed with truth in word, and faith of deed;
> Ready of wit, and fearing nought but shame:
> If that be sin, which in fixt hearts doth breed
> A loathing of all loose unchastity:
> Then love is sin, and let me sinful be!   — xiv.

This is love on the high platonic, as well as high human, level, in the spirit of Michelangelo's lines, or Donne's tribute to the Countess of Bedford —

> Madam,
> You have refined me, and to worthiest things.

But as often Sidney's mood is the rebellious appeal —

O give my passions leave to run their race !

The influence of Stella, of the "Star," is that of the radiant stars which Michelangelo describes. In sonnets lxi, lxii, she makes her own "sweet breathed defence" —

That who indeed infelt affection bears,
So captives to his saint both soul and sense;
That wholly hers, all selfness he forbears:
Thence his desires he learns, his life's course thence.

The term "saint" was peculiarly affected by the adherents of the "new religion in love," as Suckling was later to dub platonism. This sublimated love Stella will reciprocate —

Late tired with woe, even ready for to pine
With rage of love, I called my love " unkind !"
She in whose eyes love, though unfelt, doth shine
Sweetly said, "That I, true love in her should find."
I joyed ; but straight thus watered was my wine.
"That love she did, but loved a love not blind;
Which would not let me, whom she loved, decline
From nobler course, fit for my birth and mind :
And therefore by her love's authority,
Willed me, these tempests of vain love to fly ;
And anchor fast myself on Virtue's shore." — lxii.

For awhile he is still rebellious.

No more ! my Dear ! no more these counsels try !
O give my passions leave to run their race ! — lxxiv.

Then, of a sudden, he ecstatically rejoices in her conditional grace —

For Stella hath with words (where faith doth shine),
Of her high heart given me the monarchy:
I! I! O I may say that she is mine.
And though she give but thus conditionally
This realm of bliss, "while virtuous course I take:"
No kings be crowned, but they some covenant make.
— lxix.

He recognizes in her the true *platonique* —

. . . not content to be perfection's heir,
Thyself doth strive all minds that way to move;
Who mark in thee, what is in thee most fair:
So while thy beauty draws the heart to love,
As fast thy virtue bends that love to good.[1] — lxxi.

"Quiet she" — like the *primum mobile*, drawing all by divine grace-giving grace; "he, passion-rent" still, but ever more subdued to

Service and Honour, Wonder with Delight,
Fear to offend, Will worthy to appear,
Care shining in mine eyes, Faith in my sprite:
These things are left me by my only Dear. — lxxii.

And as reward for their observance, the sacra-
mental kiss is bestowed —

[1] The function of the "society" platonique of the period
was twofold: (1) to influence, through intimate relations, a
particular servant; (2) to diffuse her influence more formally
through a coterie of "servants." Lady Rich fulfilled both
functions: besides having her "*chevalier intime*," Sidney,
she received poetic incense from a coterie of Elizabethan
writers. R. Barnfield dedicated to her his *Affectionate*

. . . Kiss ! which souls, even souls together ties
By links of love. . . .   — lxxxi.

In this realization of Castiglione's like-justified
reward is the climax of the sonnet-drama, at least
as posthumously published. The rest is com-
plaint for misunderstandings, absence, sickness,
and the ever outbreaking of the lover's lower self ;
until at last he despairs. But the sequence is
manifestly on Petrarchan lines, and Petrarch ends
in reconcilement with self, and with God; so
we may well regard two other famous sonnets by
Sidney as intended for the epilogue to his sonnet-
drama.[1] In the first, apostrophizing Desire, he
protests to have at last overcome its baleful
power ; in the second, he rises above even purified
love of mortal beauty to the love of the divine
"elements" themselves of beauty, in God. The
two sonnets at once round up the dramatic sequence by the triumph of Stella, the star of love,
seen first as Woman, then as God, and epitomize
the platonic principle of evolution at its highest.
I therefore venture to quote them, familiar as they
are.

Shepherd (1594), as a "meane offering" to her "Iuorie
Shrine:" Bartholomew Yong dedicated to her his transla-
tions, both of Montemayor's *Diana* and of Guazzo's *Civile
Conversazione*, Book IV; John Davies of Hereford and
Henry Constable addressed sonnets to her.

[1] Cf. also Lee, *op. cit.*, p. xlvi.

M

Thou blind man's mark ! thou fool's self-chosen snare !
Fond fancy's scum ! and dregs of scattered thought !
Band of all evils ! cradle of causeless care !
Thou web of will ! whose end is never wrought.
    Desire ! Desire ! I have too dearly bought,
With price of mangled mind, thy worthless ware !
Too long ! too long asleep thou hast me brought !
Who should my mind to higher things prepare ;
    But yet in vain, thou hast my ruin sought !
In vain, thou mad'st me to vain things aspire !
In vain, thou kindlest all thy smoky fire !
For virtue hath this better lesson taught.
    Within myself, to seek my only hire :
    Desiring nought, but how to kill Desire.

Leave me, O love ! which reachest but to dust !
And thou, my mind ! aspire to higher things !
Grow rich in that, which never taketh rust !
Whatever fades, but fading pleasure brings.
    Draw in thy beams, and humble all thy might
To that sweet yoke, where lasting freedoms be !
Which breaks the clouds, and opens forth the light
That doth both shine, and give us sight to see.
    O take fast hold ! Let that light be thy guide !
In this small course which birth draws out to death :
And think how evil becometh him to slide,
Who seeketh heaven, and comes of heavenly breath !
    Then farewell, world ! Thy uttermost I see !
    Eternal Love, maintain Thy love in me !

It may be conceded that, as Mr. Lee insists,
both of these sonnets have an "imitative quality."
Of the joint theme of both, one prototype among

many is thus translated by George Santayana
from Lorenzo de' Medici —

> As a lamp, burning through the waning night,
> When the oil begins to fail that fed its fire
> Flares up, and in its dying waxes bright
> And mounts and spreads the better to expire;
> So in this pilgrimage and earthly flight
> The ancient hope is spent that fed desire,
> And if there burn within a greater light
> 'Tis that the vigil's end approacheth nigher.
> Hence thy last insult, Fortune, cannot move,
> Nor death's inverted torches give alarm;
> I see the end of wrath and bitter moan.
> My fair Medusa into sculptured stone
> Turns me no more, my Siren cannot charm.
> Heaven draws me up to its supernal love.[1]

Mr. Santayana speaks of thought here rising
"to the purest sphere of tragedy and of religion."
Assuredly, the same comment may be passed upon
Sidney's "thought." Neither as mere clever
jeux d'esprit of an Italianate *virtuoso*, nor as the
chronique scandaleuse, moving but shameless, of
an Elizabethan Châteaubriand, were the sonnets
of Astrophel to Stella felt by Sidney's contemporaries; but as rising "to the purest sphere of
tragedy and of religion." The silliness of Renaissance platonic love as a fad and fancy of
cynical beaux and brainless coquettes was as

[1] *Poetry and Religion*, New York, 1900, p. 135.

patent to our ancestors as to ourselves: many before John Cleveland similarly counselled such "Platonicks" —

> For shame, thou everlasting wooer. . . .
> For shame, you pretty female elves,
> Cease thus to candy up yourselves !

But Castiglione's serenely dignified gentleman was no candified fop; if anything, he might prove a little over-serious, a little of a "mollycoddle," in these days. The sixteenth century produced two notable incarnations of him in his religious love — the old Michelangelo and the young Sidney. Both — but one in beautiful, sad serenity, the other after struggle and fever — are able at last to say to the lady of their ideal : —

> Beata l' alma ove non corre tempo
> Per te s' è fatta a contemplare Dio.

> (Blessed the soul where runs no longer time
> By thee empowered to contemplate God.)

If Penelope Devereux could so "empower" at the last Sidney, we can well understand with M. Jusserand how she, "in spite of her faults, more and more visible, in spite of her far from exemplary life, remained, for the friends of the Muses, a sacred and semi-divine being, for no other reason than that she had been Sidney's love." Only, this "love" we must understand as Sidney's contemporaries understood it, and *not* according to "the critics of three hundred years later." And furthermore, if we are to take Sidney at his word at all, we should assuredly take him at his own word, and not according to our opinion of what a twentieth-century man would have done or said in his place. It is grossly unhistorical to dismiss an ideal as silly or prurient three centuries ago, because it became so later. Of course, Sidney may be lying to conceal an adulterous adventure, or — to speak more euphemistically — feigning. There is no disputing about the *possibility* of a fact; and — to repeat another truism — while there is imagination, there is doubt. But at least the burden of proof is on the doubter; and he will, I surmise, find it a hard task to rebut the actual evidence in Sidney's character, notably serious and chivalrous — "the president of nobleness and chevalree" [1] — capable of fanatic devotion to an idea, in the contemporary conception of him as the "right courtier" of Castiglione's stamp, and in the contemporary unambiguous exaltation of his love for "Stella" as of the "new religion in love."

[1] Spenser, *Shep. Cal. Præmium.*

PRÉCIEUSES AT THE COURT OF CHARLES I

THE Court of James I, less licentious than that of his grandson, Charles II, was far grosser. James himself set the tone of brutal crudity of speech and manners. The notorious orgy at the Entertainment at Theobald's to Christian of Denmark in 1606 may be an extreme, but is by no means an uncharacteristic, illustration of the grossness of the times. Nor was Sir John Harington, to whose graphic letter we owe knowledge of the orgy, a Puritan. On the contrary, about fifteen years earlier he had been disciplined by Elizabeth for certain scabrous writings of his own. But these had been at least partially redeemed by wit, whereas the gayeties at Theobald's were merely bestial. His letter to Mr. Secretary Barlow [1] is well known, and need not be transcribed here. Certainly, after perusing it, one sympathizes with the regretful comment of the disgusted gentleman: "I have much marveled at these strange pageantries, and they do bring to my remem-

[1] *Nug. Antiq.*, London, 1804, I, 348 seq.

brance what passed of this sort in our Queen's days; of which I was sometime an humble presenter and assistant: but I ne'er did see such lack of good order, discretion, and sobriety as I have now done." Later in the same remarkable letter, speaking more generally: "I will now, in good sooth, declare to you, who will not blab, that the gunpowder fright [1] is got out of all our heads, and we are going on, hereabouts, as if the devil was contriving every man should blow up himself, by wild riot, excess and devastation of time and temperance. The great ladies do go well-masked, and indeed it be the only show of their modesty, to conceal their countenance; but alack they meet with such countenance to uphold their strange doings, that I marvel not at ought that happens." The need of some refining influence at court was obvious and urgent.

Naturally, courtiers like Harington, gentlemen at bottom, might have looked to the ladies of the court for such a refining influence. And, if the consensus of poets may be trusted, among these others, masked courtesans in the derived as well as primitive meaning of the word, there were not wanting women of fine breeding and high-toned feeling. The Queen, Anne of Denmark, seems herself to have been a worthy woman, "generally

[1] The Gunpowder Plot, 1605.

well wished:" [1] as the phrase in the time ran.
The Lady Arabella Stuart wrote of her in 1603: [2]
". . . if ever thear weare such a vertu as curtesy
at the Court, I marvell what is becom of it, for
I protest I see little or none of it but in the Queene,
etc." Anne appears, however, to have been
something of a cypher at court. Of the rest,
Lucy Harrington, Countess of Bedford, unques-
tionably from her house at Twickenham exer-
cised the widest refining influence. Enthusiastic
testimonies to her are to be found in the works
of Donne, Drayton, Ben Jonson, Samuel Daniel,
and others. In Donne's *Verse-Epistles* to her,
especially, there are forehints of the platonizing
cult which is to become explicit in the next generation. "Madam," he exclaims: —

You have refined me, and to worthiest things —
Virtue, art, beauty, fortune.

In another *Epistle* more generally: —

You, or your virtue, two vast uses serves;
It ransoms one sex, and one court preserves.

That Donne may have had in mind the Italianate doctrine of platonic, or rather neo-platonic,

[1] Scandal in Scotland, to be sure, had associated her name
with Murray's.
[2] J. Nichols: *The Progresses*, etc., *of King James I.*, London, 1828, I, 265.

love,[1] is suggested by the apparent allusion in the following *Epistle* to the "myth of the cave" in Plato's *Republic*, Bk. VII.   Donne is addressing Catharine Howard, Countess of Salisbury; he has compared her to a book in which all wisdom and virtue may be learned, and adds: —

> Nor lack I light to read this book, though I
> In a dark cave, yea, in a grave do lie;
> For as your fellow-angels, so you do,
> Illustrate them who come to study you.

Other great ladies might be named, who in their own lives and circles more or less publicly rebuked the indecent coarseness of court manners; but during James's lifetime, another personal trait of the Scottish "Solomon" militated against any sway at court of feminine influences, except those which pandered to "the brutal sex." James himself despised women almost as cordially as he did tobacco, and rarely lost an opportunity of insulting them.   Above all, women who aspired to control men enraged him.   Ben Jonson caters to this mood in his *Masque of the Metamorphosed Gipsies*, 1621, in a kind of mock-litany.   Patrico intones: —

[1] Systematically expounded by Card. Bembo, Castiglione's mouthpiece in *Il Cortegiano*, Book IV.   It is virtually a sermon on the text: "The end of desire is the beginning of wisdom," applied specifically to love.   Cf. Rosi, *Saggio sui Trattati d'Amore del Cinquecento*, 1899.

> From . . .
> A smock rampant and the itches
> To be putting on the breeches —
> Wheresoe'er they have their being, . . .

And the chorus responds : —

> Bless the sovereign and his Seeing.

Toward the end of James's life, his well-known antipathy to women who aspired beyond the household seems to have led to a sort of anti-feminist crusade. A letter of 1619–1620 records: "Our pulpits ring continually of the insolence and impudence of women; and to help forward, the players have likewise taken them to task, and so to the ballads and ballad-singers, so that they can come nowhere but their ears tingle. And if all this will not serve, the King threatens to fall upon their husbands, parents, or friends, that have or should have power over them, and make them pay for it." [1]

[1] Nichols, *op. cit.*, III, 588. Mr. Chamberlain to Sir Dudley Carleton. An instance of this prying of the King into the domestic business of his subjects is recorded in Nichols, *op. cit.*, III, 529. The same Chamberlain writes to the same Carleton: "The King was pleased with his (Sir George Calvert's) answer and modesty, and sending for him, asked many questions, most about his wife. His answer was, that she was a good woman, and had brought him ten children; and would assure his Majesty, that she was not a wife with a witness. This and some other passages of this kind seem to show that the King is in a great vein of taking down high-handed women."

James was a sentimental man,[1] as gushing
letters to his "master-mistresses," Carr and
Villiers, amply prove; he was a doting father,
but he rarely vouchsafed a tender word to any
woman. His son, Charles, however, united with
his father's sentimentality a romantic passion
for women in general, and for his French wife
in particular, which made possible the taunt of
his enemies later that he was "women-led."
Whatever cold policy may have actuated Buck-
ingham, Charles's attitude in the famous *opera
bouffe* quest of the Spanish *Infanta* was that of a
young knight errant. Nor was Charles, like his
son, ever cynical in his gallantries. He is said to
have blushed like a girl at coarse language. He
had many quarrels with the capriciously way-
ward Henrietta Maria, mainly from jealousy of
other women's influence over her; but no serious charge has ever been made, even by his
Puritan enemies, against Charles's character as
a husband, unless, indeed, that already mentioned
of uxoriousness.

Under such a sovereign, delicate morally and
physically, romantic in temperament and reading, deferentially in love with a beautiful, im-

[1] An effeminate man, also, as proved by his contemporary
agnomen of "Queen James," in contradistinction to "King
Elizabeth."

perious woman, his wife, it is evident that the
whole tenor of the court was instantly altered.
Women, headed by the Queen and her intimate
Lucy Percy, Countess of Carlisle, at once assumed
direction of court life; and certainly, whatever
distresses the impetuous daughter of Henry of
Navarre may, by her political intermeddling,
have brought upon the English people, her influence toward the refining of manners in a people
sorely in need thereof was potent, and, if in some
things paradoxical, excellent. The specific tone
of Henrietta Maria's refinement imposed by her
upon the English court was naturally that to
which she had herself been attuned in France:
she was a *Précieuse.* She had been a little girl
of six when in 1615 the Marquise de Rambouillet
established her celebrated *salon* in direct protest
against crudities of speech and conduct at court
comparable to those of the contemporary court
of James I. The formative years of the future
Queen, therefore, had been subject to the con-
genial influences of the Hôtel de Rambouillet
before that had degenerated by aggravation of
mannerism and purism into the butt of Molière's
ridicule. The reforms of the Hôtel were directed
principally toward two ends — the purification
of the language and of the relations between the
sexes, and its code-book in both matters was the

preciously written love-encyclopedia in the form of a novel, *L'Astrée*, of Honoré D'Urfé's.

L'Astrée illustrates all types of love from the Don Juan-like lustful inconstancy of Hylas to the immaculate platonism of the doctrinaire Silvandre, who expounds once more the doctrine of Castiglione's Bembo and of Marguerite of Navarre's Dagoucin.[1]

It is difficult nowadays not to take the idea of so-called "platonic love" humorously. We generally regard it as something "either very silly or very dangerous."[2]   Under the paradox, however, there lies, I think, an ideal very deep and very permanent which has variously, but always potently, affected human history.   It is an ideal peculiarly feminine, for it has been woman always who has resented most bitterly the animal element in human love, and has urged most passionately the power and duty of higher natures to love without desire.   It was this aspiration which led medieval nun and monk to mystic espousal

---

[1] Between Castiglione and D'Urfé, platonic love had sporadic revivals both in France and England.   In France, Maurice Scève and the Lyons coterie about him took it seriously (*cf.* the *Revue d'Histoire Littéraire de la France*, 1896, III. 1 *sq.*) ; in England Spenser and Sidney likewise, although not so radically.

[2] So A. W. Ward: *Hist. Eng. Dram. Lit.*, ed. 1899, III. 170.

with the Christ, or with the Mother of Christ;
which moved the knightly troubadour to a loving
service of an inaccessible dame, in which no reward was asked but the right to serve; which,
later, in the revived paganism of the Renaissance,
found new sanction in the supposed doctrine of
Plato's *Banquet*, according to which grosser man
is led upward from the contemplation of woman's
beautiful person to the contemplation of the truer
beauty of her mind and soul, and thence to the
Beauty which is God. Even in more modern
times, it is immaculate loving which is the pith
of Wagner's Parsifal, whose one visible conquest
is over desire.

Of course, it is easy to paint the obverse of the
medal. Immaculate love, it may be said, is an
ideal not above, but against, nature. This view
has, perhaps, never been stated better than by
the courtly pastoralist, Guarini, in the warning by
the old shepherd Linco, in *Il Pastor Fido* to the
young Silvio, who scoffs at the power of desire.

> Uomo sono, e mi pregio
> D' essere umano; e teco, che sei uomo,
> O che piuttosto esser dovresti, parlo
> Di cosa umana: e se di cotal nome
> Forse ti sdegni, guarda
> Che nel disumanarti
> Non diventi una fera, anzi che un Dio.[1]

[1] Julie in Mrs. Humphry Ward's novel, *Lady Rose's Daughter*, Chap. XXIII, makes the same reflection upon the platonic

The justification of that warning is the history of asceticism, of chivalric love,[1] of platonic love.[2] But as Professor William James has so admirably argued in his *Varieties of Religious Belief*, religious experiences — and the aspiration to an immaculate love is surely a religious experience — are ultimate personal facts, incommensurable with all but like experiences. The historical test is after all fallacious. To know the ideal of asceticism, we should probe, not the records of the Dissolution of the Monasteries, but the mind of St. Catherine of Siena; to understand chivalric love, we should not look for the rake under the Provençal troubadour, but for the saint in Dante; so, to see what is not "either very silly or very dangerous" in platonic love, it is not to the disgusting *cicisbeo* of the eighteenth century that we should turn, but to a Michelangelo.

The phase of platonic love, however, which the young Henrietta Maria was certainly instru-

quixotism of her husband, who "seemed to her perhaps less than man, in being more."

[1] Cf. Lecky, *Hist. Europ. Morals*, ed. N. Y., 1867, II, 367; W. A. Neilson, *The Court of Love*, Harvard Studies and Notes, 1899; L. F. Mott, *The System of Courtly Love*, Diss. Columbia, 1896.

[2] The history of the degeneration of Renaissance "platonic love" into "*Cicisbeismo*" is, so far as I know, yet to be written. It is an unsavory, yet highly significant, chapter of social history.

mental in making fashionable at the English
Court, seems to incline, I fear, rather to the silly
and dangerous side than to the sublime; yet I
should not venture to assert that none of its adherents took it seriously or nobly. At any
rate, it considerably affected English manners
and English letters, and for that reason, whatever
its moral worth, demands attention. That there
was a fashion of platonic love at court about
1630 is well known; but its bearing on life and
letters has, I believe, hardly been investigated.
All that the present essay can pretend, is to open
up the matter and present a few literary data in
connection.

The chief documentary evidence of the fashion as such is in a letter written from Westminster,
June 3, 1634, by James Howell to a friend in
Paris: "The Court affords little News at present,
but that there is a Love called *Platonic Love*,
which much sways thereof late; it is a Love abstracted from all corporeal gross Impressions
and sensual Appetite, but consists in Contempla-
tions and Ideas of the Mind, not in any carnal
Fruition. This Love sets the Wits of the Town
on work; and they say there will be a Mask
shortly of it, whereof Her Majesty, and her Maids
of Honour, will be part."[1]   That the fashion lasted

---

[1] J. Howell, *Letters*, ed. London, 1754, p. 255.

is further evidenced by the same writer in a letter of February 2, 1637: "*F. C.* Soars higher and higher every Day in Pursuance of his *Platonic Love*; but *T. Man* is out with his, you know whom; he is fallen into that Averseness to her, that he swears he would rather see a Basilisk than her."[1]

The "Mask" to which Howell alludes is almost certainly Sir William D'Avenant's *The Temple of Love*, set by Inigo Jones, and acted by the Queen and her ladies at Whitehall on Shrove-Tuesday, 1634. D'Avenant himself declares that this Masque, "for the newness of the invention, variety of scenes, apparitions, and richness of habits was generally approved to be one of the most magnificent that hath been done in England." It certainly must have furthered the cause of platonic love, since in it the Queen is explicitly declared the founder of that "new religion in love."

> Who shall bring this mischief to our art?

asks one of three Magicians in the Anti-Masque. "Our art" is the art of love in the Ovidian sense. Another Magician answers: —

> Indamora,[2] the delight of destiny!

[1] *Ibid.*, p. 396. Cf. James Shirley in *The Lady of Pleasure*, V, i. Acted 1635 (Ward).

[2] *I.e.* Queen Henrietta Maria.

N

> She, and the beauties of her train ; who sure
> Though they discover Summer in their looks,
> Still carry frozen Winter in their blood.
> They raise strange doctrines, and new sects of Love
> Which must not woo or court the person, but
> The mind ; and practice generation not
> Of bodies but of souls. . . .

To the question,

> But where shall this new sect be planted first ?

Answer is made,

> In a dull northern isle they call Britaine.

Whereto the comment, as if Italy had not started
the doctrine : —

> Indeed, 'tis a cold northerly opinion. . . .
> . . . It will be long enough ere it
> Shall spread and prosper in the South !   Or if
> The Spaniard or Italian ever be
> Persuaded. . . .

The initiative evidently came from the court
ladies, for

> Certain young Lords at first disliked the philosophy
> As most uncomfortable, sad and new ;
> But soon inclin'd to a superior vote,
> And are grown as good Platonical lovers
> As are to be found in an hermitage, where he
> That was born last reckons above fourscore.

Sir Will D'Avenant was not among the converts

himself.   In the Prologue to his later play, *The Platonick Lovers*, acted by His Majesty's servants at the Blackfriars, 1636, he remarks with some humor : —

'Tis worth my smiles to think what enforc'd ways
And shifts, each poet hath to help his Plays.
Ours now believes the Title needs must cause,
From the indulgent Court, a kind applause,
Since there he learnt it first, and had command
T'interpret what he scarce doth understand.

Howell and D'Avenant both speak as if the fashion were a novelty in 1634.   Possibly, we may understand them to mean that it had by that time become widespread at court.   Certainly, in Jonson's *The New Inn*, which proved a flat failure in 1629, the doctrine is in full evidence ; [1] and there is interesting indication of the originators of the "new Love" at least in Jonson's own opinion.   Lady Frances Frampul is a typical Platonique, a "most Socratic lady," whose "humour" is, in Jonson's words, to think "nothing a felicity, but to have a multitude of servants,[2] and be called mistress by them."   In the regu-

[1] Probably the trouble was the intolerably tedious fooling of the comic characters, rather than the main theme.   Jonson was failing.

[2] The context of the play shows that "servants" is used in its common secondary sense of servants-in-love — *cavalieri serventi*.

lation "Court of Love," presided over by the
maid Prudence,[1] Lovell (*i.e.* Love-well), after
being sworn, oddly, on Ovid's *De Arte Amandi*,
expounds in a set speech the "new Love," namely,
that

> The end of love, is to have two made one
> In will, and in affection, that the minds
> Be first inoculated, not the bodies, etc.

Lady Frances, who has hitherto been scornful
of Lovell, is overcome by his eloquent exposition
of her preferred doctrine, and exclaims : —

> O speak, and speak for ever ! let mine ear
> Be feasted still, and filled with this banquet !
> No sense can ever surfeit on such truth,
> It is the marrow of all lover's tenets !
> Who hath read Plato, Heliodore, or Tatius,
> Sydney, D'Urfé, or all Love's fathers, like him ?
> He's there the Master of the Sentences,
> Their school, their commentary, text, and gloss,
> And breathes the true divinity of love !

Evidently, Lady Frances is a *Femme Savante*
as well as a *Précieuse*, that she thus familiarly
refers to the Greek philosopher, two Greek ro-
mancers, and the scholastic Peter Lombard,
besides the up-to-date D'Urfé. The significant
omission of Castiglione and other Italian exponents
of the doctrine, suggests, however, that the Eng-

[1] Act III, sc. ii.

lish rehabilitation of it at this time came direct
from France and D'Urfé.[1]

Courtly platonic love manifested itself in certainly three types, — possibly more, for I am not
concerned to be systematic.   There was the *salon*
type, in which a great lady dispensed her beneficent influence (and her hospitality) to a coterie
of "servants" who in turn "immortalized" her
in verse, or in dedications or in letters (which
usually sooner or later found their way into print),
or at least amused her busy idleness with *précieux
entretiens d'amour*.   Scarcely a poet of the time
but has his packet of such mock-amorous lauda-
tions ; the letters even of the sensible cosmopolite
James Howell are full of the doctrinal amourism
and precious phraseology in vogue.   Here is a
part of one to Lady Elizabeth Digby.   "Madam:
It is no improper Comparison, that a thankful
Heart is like a Box of precious Ointment, which
keeps the Smell long after the Thing is spent.
Madam (without Vanity be it spoken) such is
my Heart to you, and such are your Favours to
me ; the strong aromatic Odour they carried with
them diffused itself thro' all the Veins of my

[1] D'Urfé's influence seems to have reached England and
Germany about simultaneously.   In 1624, twenty-nine lords
and ladies of Germany formed an *Académie des Vrais Amants*,
and indited a flattering letter to D'Urfé as the only veritable
Celadon.

Heart, especially thro' the left Ventricle, where the most Illustrious Blood lies; so that the Perfume of them remains still fresh within me, and is like to do, while that Triangle of Flesh dilates and shutes itself within my Breast: Nor doth this Perfume stay there, but as all Smells naturally tend upwards, it hath ascended to my Brain," etc., etc. We may agree that something has indeed ascended to the poor man's brain. The bit is characteristic of the general infelicitous "felicity" of English *préciosité*.

This *salon* type of platonic love was, of course, the most open, being frankly impersonal, a system where an indefinite number of satellites revolve around a central life-giving (often *living*-giving) "she-sun." Lady Frances Frampul in Jonson's *The New Inn* is, before she succumbs to her "principal servant," Lovell, perfectly representative of this type. Indeed, Lovell's "character" of her in the first act very closely resembles the "Character" of a real and principal salon-leader of the time, Lucy Percy, Countess Carlisle, who was celebrated by all the cavalier poets and the French Voiture, who dominated the Queen, and in succession Strafford, and Pym. Lady Frances Frampul, says Lovell, —

. . . is

A noble lady, great in blood and fortune,

Fair and a wit! but of so bent a phant'sy,
As she thinks nought a happiness, but to have
A multitude of servants: and to get them,
Though she be very honest, yet she ventures
Upon these precipices, that would make her
Not seem so, to some prying narrow natures. . . .
She
                              . . . professeth still,
To love no soul or body, but for ends,
Which are her sports, etc.

So Lady Carlisle, according to Sir Toby,[1] will "freely discourse of love, and hear both the fancies and powers of it: but if you will needs bring it within knowledge, and boldly direct it to herself, she is likely to divert the discourse; or, at least, seem not to understand it. By which you may know her humor, and her justice; for, since she cannot love in earnest, she would have nothing from love: so contenting herself to play with *Love*, as with a child. . . . She more willingly allows of the conversation of men, than of women. . . . She is more esteem'd than belov'd by her own sex, in two respects; the one, for that her beauty far exceeds theirs; and the other, for that her wit doth the like. . . . She is so great a lover of variety, as that when she may not other-

[1] *A Collection of Letters made by Sir Tobie Mathews, Kt. with a Character of the most excellent Lady Lucy, Countesse of Carleile,* etc.   London, 1660.

wise express it, she will remove her own thoughts, if not change her opinions, even of those persons that are not least consider'd by her: and when they have given her this entertainment, let them settle again in their former places with her. . . . She believeth nothing to be worthy of her consideration but her own imagination. These gallant fancies keep her in satisfaction, when she is alone: where she will make something worthy of her liking, since, in the world she cannot find anything worthy of her loving," etc. Certainly, Lady Carlisle might have sat for Lady Frances Frampul, whether she did or not.

A second type of platonic love was where two only were involved, but where the poetical wooing was a kind of "open letter" of compliment. The language of the lover was seemingly passionate, but far less was meant than met the ear. A case of this type is, I think, the famous wooing of "Sacharissa," Lady Dorothy Sidney, by the poet Edward Waller. Waller's poems to "Sacharissa" — name, says Dr. Johnson, "derived from Sugar, and implies a spiritless mildness and dull good nature " [1] — range from about 1634 to 1638,

[1] The English *Précieux* and *Précieuses* seem also to have been familiarly known by pastoral nicknames, even in private and every-day life. Lady Carlisle was commonly known as *Aminta*. Even in a totally serious family letter, her brother, Henry Percy, calls her so, and refers to himself as *Aurelius* —

coinciding, therefore, with the height of the platonizing fashion. That Waller's wooing verse was a service in the "new religion in love" is certainly suggested by the fact that his name is never even mentioned by Lady Leicester in her frank letters to her husband among the several other suitors, by no means all welcome; and that he remained on cordial, visiting relations with the whole family, when had his wooing been serious as it was outspoken, it must have compromised the young lady. Considering these, and other facts, notably the most singular letter of congratulation written by him on Dorothy's marriage, I think there can be no reasonable doubt[1] of the "platonic" nature of this famous affair.

The third type of platonic love is hardly distinguishable, except in the special color of its philosophical jargon, from that of troubadour or minnesinger. A precise case[2] of it is to be found

whether after the Roman emperor, or from a character in the *Commedia dell' Arte*. Such nicknames were sometimes for disguise, of course, as in Sir Kenelm Digby's *Private Memoirs*.

[1] Cf. Julia Cartwright, *Sacharissa*, London, 1893.

[2] In Sir Tobie Mathew's Letter-book there is a long series of letters indicating a similar relation, but less intense, between "a great Lady" and "a most humble Servant." They are, however, too carefully guarded and pruned to be very significant. Sir Tobie's intention is to publish a "polite letter-writer," rather than to illustrate history.

in a set of letters addressed to a certain "Aglaura" by the poet Sir John Suckling.[1]   One may draw up from these letters, few as they are, almost a code-book of platonic love like that by Andreas Capellanus of chivalric love. The first in the series touches the primary article of *Constancy*, with a curious permissive exception: the inconstant platonic lover is justified if he leave a lesser beauty for a greater, because beauty is in the cult the *primum mobile* of virtue. Coming to town, Suckling finds Aglaura gone; yet he writes, "though you have left behind you faces whose beauties might well excuse perjury in others, yet in me they cannot, since to the making that no sin casuists have most rationally resolved that she for whom we forsake ought to be handsomer than the forsaken, which would be here impossible." *His service is its own reward:* "after all, the wages will not be high, for it (his heart) hath been brought up under Platonics, and knows no other way of being paid for service than by being commanded more." *Her virtue's will is his will:* he promises, therefore, to forego his pet vice of gambling; but humorously adds, "since I know your ladyship is too wise to suppose to yourself impossibilities, and therefore cannot think of such a thing as of making me absolutely good, it will not

[1] *Works*, London, 1874, II, pp. 178 *et seq.*

be without some impatience that I shall attend to
know what sin you will be pleased to assign me
in the room of this." He protests his *humility*,
and considers "that I have no pretence to your
favours than that which all men have to the original of beauty, light, which we enjoy, not that
'tis the inheritance of our eyes, but because things
most excellent cannot restrain themselves, but
are ours, as they are diffusively good." He
exalts *purity*, while deprecating his own frailty:
"though desire, in those that love, be still like
too much sail in a storm, and man cannot so easily
strike, or take all in when he pleases; yet dearest
princess, be it never so hard, when you shall think
it dangerous, I shall not make it difficult; though
— well, love is love, and air is air; and though
you are a miracle yourself, yet do I not believe
that you can work any." [1] Upon this more
intimate type of platonic love, as in chivalric love,
secrecy is enjoined: "though I can never be

[1] In his play called *Aglaura*, acted before 1638, Suckling
makes a character ask: —

> . . . Shall souls refined not know
> How to preserve alive a noble flame,
> But let it die — burn out to appetite?

To which Semanthe, "a Platonic," replies: —

> Love's a chameleon and would live on air,
> Physic for agues; starving is his food.

ashamed to be found an idolater to such a shrine
as yours, yet since the world is full of profane
eyes, the best way sure is to keep all mysteries
from them, and to let privacy be (what indeed
it is) the best part of devotion." [1] In another
letter, to a "Lord," Suckling intimates that the
code was being occasionally violated, and suggests
also a perilous line of casuistry. After dwelling
on the reformation in morale at Charles's court,
he adds with irony: "to be a little pleasant in
my instances: the very women have suffered
reformation, and wear through the whole court
their faces as little disguised now as an honest
man's actions should be; [2] and if there be any
suffered themselves to be gained by their servants,
their ignorance of what they granted may well
excuse them from the shame of what they did."

[1] Cf. Donne's

> 'Twere profanation of our joys
> To tell the laity our love.

And William Habington's *To a friend inquiring her name,
whom he loved:* —

> 'Twere prophanation of my zeale,
> If but abroad one whisper steale,
> They love betray who him reveale.

[2] Cf. Harington's gibe at the fashion of masks, *supra*,
p. 121.

I suppose he affects to believe that as love-mystics, their tranced souls were oblivious to the acts of their irrelevant bodies.[1]

Such are the main types of platonic love in the fashion.   The literature on the theme ranges in mood all the way from exalted mysticism through mere gallantry to mocking cynicism.   The mystics of the "new religion in love" talk of ecstasies directly in line with the religious ἔχστασις of Plotinus.   The model of this kind is Donne's *Ecstasy*, which, although earlier, is too pertinent to pass by. The poem opens with completest mystic exaltation.

> . . . our souls negotiate there,
>   We like sepulchral statues lay ;
> All day, the same our postures were,
>   And we said nothing all the day.

---

[1] John Cleveland humorously exculpates an erring Quaker on the same ground : —

> 'Twas but an Insurrection
> Of the Carnal Part,
>   For a Quaker in Heart
> Can never lose Perfection.
> For so our Matters teach us,
> The Intent being well directed,
>   Though the Devil trapan
>   The Adamical Man,
> The Saints stand uninfected.
>   *Works*, London, 1687, p. 338.

This communion of souls was pure and purifying:

> If any, so by love refined,
>   That he souls' language understood,
> And by good love were grown all mind,
>   Within convenient distance stood,
>
> He — though he knew not which soul spake,
>   Because both meant, both spake the same —
> Might thence a new concoction take,
>   And part far purer than he came.

The ecstasy transcends sex: —

> This ecstasy doth unperplex
>   (We said) and tell us what we love;
> We see by this, it was not sex, etc.

Rather, perhaps, applying Socrates' fantasy of sundered half bodies seeking reunion to sundered lonely half souls, Donne conceives these as by "elective affinity" compounded in the ecstasy to a third soul self-sufficient, immortal: —

> When love with one another so
>   Interanimates two souls,
> That abler soul, which thence doth flow,
>   Defects of loneliness controls.
>
> We then, who are this new soul, know,
>   Of what we are composed and made,
> For th' atomies of which we grow
>   Are souls, whom no change can invade.

Then follows the argument that this quintessential union of souls is attainable only through the prior initiation of bodies : —

> So must pure lovers' souls descend
>   To affections, and to faculties,
> Which sense may reach and apprehend,
>   Else a great prince in prison lies.
>
> To our bodies turn we then, that so
>   Weak men on love reveal'd may look;
> Love's mysteries in souls do grow,
>   But yet the body is his book.

Donne is probably nearer here to Plato than the *Précieuses* ever were; but the love-philosophy of these wholly repelled any such rehabilitation of "gross corporeal Impressions." Accordingly, Donne's disciple, Lord Herbert of Cherbury, as a consistent *Précieux*, in his obvious imitation of the *Ecstasy*, *An Ode upon a question moved whether Love should continue forever*,[1] emasculates Donne to conformity with courtly feminist propriety. His entranced pair have the refined names, Melander and Celinda. The tone of their love-debate is of languishing sensibility. They are all soul, and as good as have no bodies. At the last,

[1] *Poems*, ed. J. Churton Collins, London, 1881, p. 92.

> . . . Such a moveless silent peace
> Did cease on their becalmed sense,
> One would have thought some Influence
> Their ravish'd spirits did possess.

This is, indeed, a situation in the "Countreys undiscovered" beyond "The Dangerous Sea" of the *"Carte du Tendre."* Lord Herbert has three other poems,[1] all entitled *Platonick Love*, and all in the same vein.[2]

If Donne's *Ecstasy* represents the virile mood of platonic love, and Herbert's the effeminate, or feminist, John Cleveland's *To Cloris, a Rapture* [3] has an evident tone of cynical irony under its irreproachable outer conformity to the code.

> Come, Julia, Come! Let's once disbody, what,
> Straight Matter ties to this, and not to that?
> We'l disingage, our bloodless Form shall fly
> Beyond the reach of Earth, where ne'er an Eye
> That peeps through Spectacles of Flesh, shall know
> Where we intend, or what we mean to do.
> From all contagion of Flesh remov'd, etc.
> . . . Thus wee'l like Angels move, nor will we bind
> In words the copious language of our Mind, etc.

[1] *Ibid.* pp. 104, 106, 114.

[2] Herbert seems to have acted out his platonic doctrine with a certain "fairest of her time." See his *Life*, London, 1826, pp. 96, 152.

[3] *Works*, London, 1687, p. 309. Carew's celebrated *Rapture* has, of course, no relation to platonic love, unless, perhaps, as deliberate reaction.

Whatever its degree of sincerity, this ecstasy of platonic love was manifestly anti-sociable. The court *Précieuses*, however, had no wish to transform Whitehall into another Palace of Sleeping Beauty, however ecstatic the sleep. In London, as in Paris, the new art of loving was in effect an art of talking about love. The Roxanes of the court desired lip-service. Lovell's eloquence of doctrine moves Lady Frances, not his constancy or passion. Jonson's *New Inn*, indeed, points to a revival of the regularization of love-debates under legal form and ceremony, as in the medieval Courts of Love. Justice Prue's "charge" is quite after Castiglione's code [1] of *ragionamenti d'amore*. She enjoins upon Lovell

> Not to give ear or admit conference
> With any person but yourself : nor there,
> Of any other argument but LOVE,
> And the companion of it, gentle courtship,
> For which your two hours' service, you shall take
> Two kisses. . . .

Castiglione had long ago ordained that the platonic lady, "*per compiacer al suo amante bono, oltre il concedergli i risi piacevoli, i ragionamenti domestici e secreti, il motteggiare, scherzare, toccar la mano, pò venir ancor ragionevolmente senza*

[1] Cf. *Il Cortegiano*, ed. Cian, Florence, 1894, Bk. III, §§ LIII -LXXIII; Bk. IV, §§ XLIX *et seq.*

o

biasimo insin al bascio, il che nel-l' amor sensuale, secondo le regule del Signor Magnifico, non e licito," etc.[1]

Besides the at least literary rehabilitation of the "courts of love,"[2] the platonizing fashion seems to have revived — of course not deliberately — the troubadour custom of disputations in verse. Thus Waller controverts[3] formally, clause by clause, a poem of Suckling's *Against Fruition.* For example, here is a specimen of the debate, as Waller prints it : —

---

[1] *Op. cit.* § LXIV.

[2] In Marston's *Parasitaster* (pr. 1606) and in Massinger's *The Parliament of Love* (acted 1624) courts of love are also introduced. Each is presided over by Cupid, however, and the point is not to provide witty discourse of love as in Jonson's, but to resolve a concrete situation of very crude love. They are neither feminist nor platonist.

During the lifetime of the chivalrous Prince Henry "questions of love" were sometimes submitted to the arbitrament of combat. See Nichols's *Progresses*, etc., *of James I,* Vol. II, pp. 49, 51, 716, 727. In the last cited, Jonson's *A Challenge at Tilt at a Marriage,* Dec. 27 and Jan. 1, 1613-1614, the question is as to the superiority in love of Man, "the nobler creature," or of Woman, "the purer." Anteros, who sustains the Woman's cause, is in another Masque, *Love Restor'd,* called by Jonson "Anti-Cupid, the Love of Virtue," and, therefore, identical with platonic love as defined by the *Précieuses.*

[3] In a poem called, *In Answer of Sir John Suckling's Verses (Against Fruition)* — Waller, *Poems,* London, 1730, p. 97.

CON (i.e. Suckling)

Women enjoy'd, whate'er before they've been,
Are like Romances read, or scenes once seen:
  Fruition dulls, or spoils the Play, much more
Than if one read, or knew, the plot before.

PRO (i.e. Waller)

Plays, and Romances read, and seen, do fall
In our opinions: yet, not seen at all,
Whom would they please? To an heroic tale
Would you not listen, lest it should grow stale?

CON

'Tis expectation makes a blessing dear;
Heav'n were not heav'n, if we knew what it were.

PRO

If 'twere not heav'n, if we knew what it were,
'Twould not be heav'n to those that now are there.

Sir William D'Avenant's *The Platonick Lovers*
is what may be called a drama of love-debate. Of
action there is almost none, the whole business of
the play being ingenious disputation for and against
fruition of love in marriage. The issue is rather
crudely presented in two pairs of lovers — Theander and Eurithea[1] who love platonically,

---

[1] The play, printed, is dedicated to Henry Jermyn, Esq.,
whose relations with Henrietta Maria had been dubiously
intimate. Eurithea is plainly the Queen. Can D'Avenant
be intending an apology?

Phylomont and Ariola, who love naturally. Although D'Avenant's own attitude is that of masculine common sense, and he lets Hymen win, yet he really does put not a little poetry into the soulful converse of the platonics, in their yet unreconstructed estate. If Theander is morbid and a *Précieux*, Phylomont is a good deal of a brute; so that Theander's rebuke to Phylomont's crude definition of natural desire may stand for the whole justification, such as it is, of the feminist paradox.

> You are too masculine!
> . . . you blast me with
> Your breath. Poor ruffians in their drink, that dwell
> In suburb alleys, and in smoky lanes
> Are not so rude.

Waller's and Suckling's epicurean considerations for or against fruition and D'Avenant's all "too masculine" insistence on the natural rite and rights of matrimony are equally hostile to any serious taking of the "cold, northerly opinion" of platonism. Lord Herbert of Cherbury was perhaps more in earnest. For the absolute platonic in heavy earnest, however, we must turn from the courtier to a Catholic gentleman of the higher middle class, William Habington.[1]

---

[1] Imitation of high life in *bourgeois* circles always accentuates what it imitates. Hence Molière, to find caricature in fact, makes his *Précieuses Ridicules* middle-class girls.

In 1635, or before, — Oldys calls this the second edition, — Habington published his *Castara*, a *canzoniere* in three parts, the first of his courtship, the second of his married life, the third of his religious life. The opening sentences of his general preface are interesting as evincing the fact that French influence was already superseding Italian, and that the literary tendencies of the moment were feminist. ". . . I never set so high a rate upon it [poetry], as to give myself entirely up to its devotion. It hath too much ayre, and (if without offence to our next transmarine neighbour) wantons too much according to the French garbe. And when it is wholly imployed in the soft straines of love, his soule who entertaines it, loseth much of that strength which should confirme him man. The nerves of judgement are weakened most by its dalliance; and when woman (I meane onely as she is externally faire) is the supreme object of wit, we soone degenerate into effeminacy. For the religion of fancie declines into a mad superstition, when it adores that idoll which is not secure from age and sicknesse. Of such heathens, our times afford us a pittyed multitude," etc. These sentiments, reflecting Bacon's contemptuous mood toward love,[1] seem an odd prelude to a collection of love-

[1] "As if Man, made for the contemplation of Heaven, and all Noble Objects, should doe nothing but kneele before a little

poems; but Habington hastens to assure us that his is no ordinary love, nor his an ordinary lady. "In all those flames in which I burnt, I never felt a wanton heate; nor was my invention ever sinister from the straite way of chastity." The preliminary prose "character" of Castara puts her into a niche by herself among Platoniques as a kind of Puritan-platonique. Unlike the real Lady Carlisle, or the feigned Lady Frampul, "she glories not in the plurality of servants, a multitude of Adorers Heaven can onely challeng; and it is impietie in her weaknesse to desire superstition from many." Rigider than the code, "she never understood the language of a kisse, but at salutation." Habington admits his heresy, yet maintains this character of a "mistris," "though the next sinod of ladies condemne this character as an heresie broacht by a precision." Indeed, Habington's wooing would appear to have been as paradoxically "platonic" as Thenot's devotion to Clorin in *The Faithful Shepherdess*, of which, in fact, some of his poems remind one.[1] Although Habington's preface protests against the Frenchi-

---

Idoll, and make himself subject, though not of the Mouth (as Beasts are) yet of the Eye; which was given him for higher purposes." — *Essayes: Of Love.*

[1] It is significant that this pastoral-morality of chastity was presented by the Queen and her ladies before the King in 1633, the height of the platonizing fashion.

fied feminism of the day, his muse is a court platonique, after all. The poem, for example, *To the World, the Perfection of Love*, is a courtly platonist doctrinal in miniature. After the scornful invocation : —

> You who are earth, and cannot rise
> Above your sense, etc.

He boasts of himself and Castara : —

> When we speak love, nor art, nor wit
>   We glosse upon :
> Our souls engender, and beget
> Ideas, which you counterfeit
>   In your dull propagation.
>
> While time seven ages shall disperse,
>   Wee'le talke of love,
> And when our tongues hold no commerse,
> Our thoughts shall mutually converse,
>   And yet the blood no rebell prove.

Herbert's Melander and Celinda, or D'Avenant's Theander and Eurithea, could no better. Even in marriage Habington pursues his paradox. He declares *To Castara upon an embrace :* —

> If not prophane, we'll say,
>   When angels close, their joys are such ;
> For we no love obey
>   That's bastard to a fleshly touch.
> Let's close, Castara, then, since thus
> We pattern angels, and they us.

Courtly gallantry is preferable to this prurient mawkishness, especially when Habington informs us in his second "character" that "A Friend — is a man. For the free and open discovery of thoughts to woman cannot passe without an over-licentious familiarity, or a justly occasion'd suspition," etc. *"Justly occasion'd?"* . . . then how about those "seven ages" of love-talk with Castara?

Cynicism, offensive from the pharisaical Habington, is lightened by gayety in Suckling. In the play, *Aglaura*, the "Antiplatonic" Orsames is recounting his experiences with the platonique Semanthe : —

I had no sooner nam'd love to her, but she
Began to talk of flames, and flames
Neither devouring nor devour'd of air
And of chameleons.
   (1 *Courtier :*) O the Platonics !
   (2 *Courtier :*) Those of the new religion in love ! Your
     Lordship's merry,
Troth, how do you like the humor on't ?
   (*Ors.:*) . . .
A mere trick to enhance the price of kisses, etc.

In a singular play first published in 1659, *Lady Alimony*, this cynical interpretation of platonism is developed systematically and at great length. The six "alimony ladies" cashiered their husbands for the wholly unambiguous service of

as many so-called "platonic confidants." The
moralist-author puts into the mouth of the "con-
fidant" Tillyvally a plea for platonic love, concluding : —

> Stol'n waters be the sweetest.

Whereupon all the ladies in unison exclaim : —

> Excellent ;
> Thou shalt be styl'd the Platonic Pythias.

The reflection upon Lady Frampul's encomium of
Lovell as a "Father" of the faith after his defence
of the Platonic love is manifest, although perhaps
coincidental. Even more satirically explicit is
the Prologue : —

> Madams, you are welcome ; though our poet show
> A severe brow, it is not meant to you.
> Your virtues, like your features, they are such,
> They neither can be priz'd not prais'd too much :
> Lov'd and admir'd wheres'ever you are known,
> Scorning to mix Platonics with your own :
> Sit with a pleasing silence, and take view
> Of forms vermillioned in another hue,
> Who make free traffic of their nuptial bed, etc.

Considering the Queen's patronage of platonic
love, it is difficult to guess when and where so
bold an arraignment of the dangerous folly could
have been acted.

The prevailing tone of the professed anti-
platonics, however, is one of satirico-comic depre-

cation, whether of the ideal love itself or of the poet's inability to live up to its tenets. Waller (*Of Love*) compares the Court to a harem in which the courtiers, like eunuchs,

> All to one female idol bend.

Charles Cotton, who can be platonic when he chooses, witnesses this of a kiss: —

> Such a kiss to be I find
> The conversation of the mind,
> And whisper of the soul;

yet inveighs against "the monstrous regiment of women": —

> By Heav'n 'tis against all nature,
> Honour and manhood, wit and sense
> To let a little female creature
> Rule on the poor account of feature,
> And thy unmanly patience
> Monstrous and shameful as her insolence.

Roistering Dick Brome resolves: —

> Reason, henceforth, not Love, shall be my guide,
> My fellow-creatures shan't be deified;
> I'll now a rebel be,
> And so pull down
> That distaff-monarchy,
> And females' fancied crown. . . .

He admits that

> If virtue or good parts could win me,
>   I'd turn Platonic, and ne'er vex
>   My soul with difference of sex.

But "Love's without Reason;" so he scoffs, and cries : —

> Nay, fie, Platonics ! still adoring
>   The fond chimeras of your brain. . . .
> Live in your humour, 'tis a curse
>   So bad, 'twere pity wish a worse. . . .
> Cashiered wooers, whose low merit
>   Could ne'er arrive at nuptial bliss,
> Turn schismatics in love, whose spirit
>   Would have none hit, 'cause they do miss. . . .

John Cleveland, in several poems called *The Anti-Platonick* and *Platonick Love*,[1] is similarly sarcastic.

> For shame, thou everlasting wooer. . . .
> For shame, you pretty female elves,
> Cease thus to candy up yourselves. . . .

He is a frank sensualist : —

> Fond Love, what dost thou mean
>   To court an idle Folly,
> Platonick Love is nothing else
>   But merely Melancholy.

Elsewhere he is unquotably specific on the theme. Suckling ironically deprecates his own unworthiness : —

[1] Ed. 1687, pp. 11, 211, 324.

> Oh that I were all soul, that I might prove
> For you as fit a love,
> As you are for an angel; for I know
> None but pure spirits are fit loves for you.
> You are all ethereal, there's in you no dross,
> Nor any part that's gross. . . .
> Thus have your raptures reach'd to that degree
> In Love's philosophy,
> That you can figure to yourself a fire
> Void of all heat, a love without desire. . . .
> But I must needs confess I do not find
> The motions of my mind
> So purified as yet . . . etc.

But the aptest lyric protest I have happened upon
is William Cartwright's *No Platonique Love.*
Here are two stanzas : —

> Tell me no more of minds embracing minds
>   And hearts exchang'd for hearts;
> That spirits spirits meet, as winds do winds,
>   And mix their subt'lest parts;
> That two unbody'd essences may kiss,
> And then, like angels, twist and feel one bliss.
>
> I was that silly thing that once was wrought
>   To practise this their love;
> I climbed from sex to soul, from soul to thought;
>   But thinking there to move,
> Headlong I rowl'd from thought to soul, and then
> From soul I lighted at the sex again.

The tenets and the untenableness of the "new
religion in love" could hardly be more pithily
stated.

Idol and doll he has made her; he has bowed
His neck before her, petted her, — and shamed.
Spreading his nets of passion, he has tamed
Her singing spirit, love-lured from the cloud;
Till she has walked beside him, humbly proud
To be his shadow while the world acclaimed,
His cheering sunshine if the world defamed,
Her own life-hunger meekly disavowed.
Under love's spell she feels herself how frail,
Her heart how wooing love's death-sweet abuse —
The fair false glamor, and the old old tale
Of tears; yet if, heart-weary, crying a truce
With love, she rends the sacred bridal veil,
Love smiles, — and bends her to his wonted use.